Reduce Your Cancer Risk

Reduce Your Cancer Risk

Twelve Steps to a Healthier Life

Barbara Boughton

Michael Stefanek, PhD

Edited by

Ted Gansler, MD

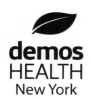

demos
HEALTH
New York

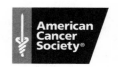

Acquisitions Editor: Noreen Henson
Cover Design: Steve Pisano
Compositor: NewGen North America
Printer: Bang Printing

Visit our website at www.demosmedpub.com

Library of Congress Cataloging-in-Publication Data

Boughton, Barbara.
    Reduce your cancer risk: twelve steps to a healthier life/Barbara Boughton, Michael Stefanek; edited by Ted Gansler.
        p. cm.
    Includes index.
    ISBN 978-1-932603-92-7
    1. Cancer—Prevention. 2. Cancer—Risk factors. I. Stefanek, Michael. II. Gansler, Ted S. III. Title.
    RC268.B68 2010
    616.99'405—dc22   2010001297

Special discounts on bulk quantities of Demos Medical Publishing books are available to corporations, professional associations, pharmaceutical companies, health care organizations, and other qualifying groups. For details, please contact:

Special Sales Department
Demos Medical Publishing
11 W. 42nd Street
New York, NY 10036
Phone: 800–532–8663 or 212–683–0072
Fax: 212–941–7842
E-mail: rsantana@demosmedpub.com

Made in the United States of America

10 11 12   13   5 4 3 2 1

This book is dedicated to my parents Anne and George, who battled breast cancer and lung cancer respectively. Thanks for showing me your bravery and generosity of spirit, for your unflagging pride in my best endeavors, and for teaching me how to persevere, to love fully, and to approach life with a sense of humor.

Barbara Boughton

With unbounded love, I dedicate my efforts on this book to my mother Mary Stefanek, a 6 year survivor of head and neck cancer, who has taught her son about courage, strength, and the incredible importance of sacrifice and giving to others. Mom, I only hope I am capable of learning your lessons and passing them on to your grandchildren.

Michael Stefanek

Contents

Preface

A Daughter's Search for Answers

The night after my mother's mastectomy, we stood at the window of her hospital room in a skyscraper and looked at the lights of Manhattan. "It's our city," she said and gave me a gentle hug. I was filled with hope, confident that we could defeat my mother's breast cancer.

But five years later, her cancer returned, and this time it had spread to her lungs and was incurable. I began to fear that cancer runs in my family, as bad teeth or allergies do in most others. My mother was only the latest in a family history that was deeply colored by the disease. From colon cancer to pancreatic cancer, lung cancers, and melanomas, both sides of my family seemed to share a distinct predisposition for the disease. Or so it seemed. I decided right then and there that I wanted to know if I was at an increased risk myself.

Perhaps you have a family or a personal history of cancer and are fearful about the disease. If so, you're not alone. Studies show that the fear of cancer is common among people with a family history of cancer. Fear of cancer is understandable in all of us, cancer history or not. But the truth is that many of us, especially those with a personal or family history of cancer, overestimate our risk for the disease, sometimes by as much as three or four times, and live with unnecessary anxiety and fear.

In one 2004 study of 400 women conducted by National Cancer Institute researchers, published in *Preventive Medicine*, women with and without a family history of breast cancer overestimated their risk for the disease by an average of 25%. Other research, published in 2000 by Duke University researchers, showed that women overestimated their risk for breast cancer by as much as 50%.

Like many people who have a family history of cancer, I once dreaded the diagnosis. At times, I wondered if I might die from this disease, just as my mother had. But gradually I came to believe that knowledge about my cancer risk and learning to face this risk head on might be my best weapon against this disease. It could help me to make a plan to prevent getting cancer in the first place and help me to deal with the fears that occasionally cropped up for me—during my annual mammogram, for instance, or when I went to my yearly dermatologist's appointment to have my moles checked for skin cancer.

The research I did about my own cancer risk helped to clear up mysteries about my family's history of cancer and helped me to devise a preventive health strategy to reduce my own exposure to the disease. In this field, information is power. Studies show that for people with a family heritage of cancer, getting accurate information about cancer risk can reduce cancer-specific worries by as much as 50%. And it certainly can help those at average risk for the disease who simply want to live a healthier life!

Through my work as a medical reporter, I was able to find out how to accurately assess my cancer risk and to make a plan that proactively addressed factors that contribute to the disease. However, you don't need to be a medical reporter to do the same. Finding out about and addressing cancer risk means taking a number of simple preventive health steps. Depending on your risk factors, this may mean visiting wellness health sites on the Internet, investigating genetic counseling, or making lifestyle choices that may significantly increase your chances for having a healthier life.

This book is divided into 12 chapters—one for each step that you can take to reduce your cancer risk. It includes information about diet, lifestyle, and the environment, as well as the genetics of cancer. It explores the many ways to modify your risk for cancer through lifestyle changes—including quitting smoking, maintaining a healthy weight, exercising, and lessening exposure to chemicals or pollutants in the environment that might cause cancer. It also explores some of the more controversial areas of cancer risk, including recent science about nutrition and cancer, dietary supplements, and complementary and alternative medicine. The chapters also include information for those at above-average risk or those who may have a genetic predisposition to cancer and delves into the areas of genetic counseling, testing, and use of medications and surgeries to prevent cancer.

But first, you may want to know, "How did I find out about my own cancer risk and learn to make a preventive health plan?" My own search for information began in 1994 with my mother's death at age 71 from breast cancer. Several years later, my mother's sister, Mary, also was diagnosed with breast cancer. Unlike my mother's cancer, though, Aunt Mary's breast cancer was caught early. But still, Aunt Mary's daughter, and my cousin, an oncologist, was concerned enough to recommend that her mother be tested for the mutations in the two breast cancer genes, *BRCA1* and *BRCA2*, that confer an elevated risk of breast and other cancers. The test results came back negative. "It means I'm not Typhoid Mary—and it's good news for you," Aunt Mary said in an early phone call to me.

I felt reassured after her phone call. It meant that the chances that I harbored a breast cancer gene were lower than I thought. At the same time, I was aware that I had an increased risk for breast cancer because of my family history. But how much risk? I first questioned my physician about my risk for breast cancer at my yearly gynecologic exam.

"Having two women in your family with breast cancer would surely mean it was genetic if they were in their 40s when the cancer was diagnosed," my physician said. "That's a true sign of inherited cancer. But both your relatives were over 60 when they first had breast cancer, and we're not sure what that means." She added, "It could be sporadic—meaning that it could have occurred twice in your family by chance—but, at the same time, we know you're at increased risk, and we have to be conscientious about getting routine screening tests, like a yearly mammogram."

I wanted to know more. I also wanted to learn about proactive health strategies that would help me to prevent cancer as best I could.

Yet I found roadblocks in the way when I delved for answers. When I searched bookstores, I discovered dozens of books about dealing with cancer or preventing it, but only three about assessing cancer risk—and one was out of print. The remaining two books concentrated exclusively on breast cancer, when my family was affected by a variety of cancers, including skin, breast, and lung cancer.

The information that I got from doctors and scientists also was contradictory. My physicians were reassuring, telling me that if I got the right screening tests, any cancer could be caught early. But, during my work on a magazine story, a researcher at the National Cancer Institute told me that a woman with two older relatives with breast cancer could have double the normal risk of getting the disease. That was frightening. What did it mean, and did those statistics apply to me?

Above all, I wanted to know if I had a high enough cancer risk to need preventive medication or a genetic test. I decided to delve deeper into the science behind cancer risk and prevention, including genetic cancer risk.

It eventually would take me to a session with a genetic counselor—a session that turned out to be tremendously reassuring and inspired me to do the initial research for this book.

*   *   *

On the day that I set out for my genetic counseling appointment, my health worries—usually pushed to the back of my mind—absorbed me. I didn't know what I would find in this venture into the world of cancer risk and genetics. Feeling decidedly irritable as I drove toward my appointment, I honked impatiently at a driver turning onto the freeway with the speed of a tortoise.

I selected my genetic counselor, Patricia Kelly, PhD, author of *Assess Your True Risk of Breast Cancer*, based on her book and experience in genetics. Her Web site noted her expertise; she is a diplomate of the American Board of Medical Genetics, a founding fellow of the American College of Medical Genetics, and has conducted research studies published in prestigious scientific journals. I had found her book informative and comprehensive, and I discovered that, lucky for me, she lived in Berkeley—just a stone's throw from my little town of El Cerrito, California.

When I got to Kelly's house, I slowly opened her garden gate. Before me was a vista that I hadn't expected—a front yard filled with colorful flowers, surrounding a winding stone path that led to the back of the house and Kelly's office. I felt a little like Alice in Wonderland.

I was early for my appointment, so I sat down in a chair in the cool entryway and drummed my fingers anxiously on a nearby table. In my lap, I precariously balanced a questionnaire that Kelly had asked me to fill out.

As I was doing research on my family history of cancer for the questionnaire, I had discovered to my chagrin that not only had my mother and her sister, Mary, had breast cancer, but my father's mother may have had the disease when she was in her 40s. I was concerned because breast cancer before age 50 may be a sign of having a hereditary disease and of having a mutation (a change or damage) in one of the breast cancer genes, *BRCA1* or *BRCA2*.

BRCA1 and *BRCA2* are thought to be tumor suppressors, helping to prevent the development of cancer. Everyone has these genes, but a mutation in one of them can result in hereditary breast cancer, as well as a greatly increased risk for ovarian cancer and a modestly increased risk for other cancers such as prostate cancer. For instance, men who carry the *BRCA1* or *BRCA2* mutations have about a 16% risk of prostate cancer by age 70, according to the National Cancer Institute.

My grandmother had entered the hospital—my father thought for breast cancer surgery—and had died of pneumonia during World War II, a time when antibiotics were not plentiful. I also found out more about other cancers on my father's side of the family. My grandfather had died of virulent pancreatic cancer, and my aunt (my father's sister) had died of cancer starting in the cecum, the section of the colon or large intestine that is closest to the small intestine. As my cousin Jane wrote to me in an e-mail, "By the time it was discovered, it was everywhere."

So I had come to this genetic counseling appointment prepared to probe further into these questions. I hoped that I would find that my risk was relatively low, but at the same time I dreaded more sobering news. Perhaps there were signs in my family's history of a genetic mutation— one that predisposed us to colon, breast, or other cancers.

Kelly arrived, a tall, thin woman with short gray hair and a shawl wrapped around her shoulders. She ushered me into her office. She spoke in a quiet, gentle, reassuring voice. I explained why I had made an appointment, and she asked me a few questions, as she peered intently at my questionnaire.

"It might be interesting for you to get a copy of your grandmother and grandfather's death records to find out more about your family history," she said. "Your grandmother's death record could probably tell you a lot. Fifty years ago, they went into a lot of detail about the reasons for death."

Then Kelly talked to me about cancer risk and showed me a picture of the size of most breast cancers found on a mammogram these days— about 1.5 cm or smaller, less than the size of a dime. "Breast cancers less than 1 cm are unlikely to recur," she said. In one study in which the breast cancers were less than 1 cm, the 16-year survival was 90%. That meant that if I ever did get breast cancer, the chances that I would survive—unlike my mother's—were pretty good. Twenty years ago, when my mother's cancer was first diagnosed, mammograms were less accurate and less often used. Most breast cancers, when diagnosed, were twice as large and more likely to recur and spread.

Kelly then informed me, to my surprise, that studies have shown that even women who have a mother and a sister with breast cancer are not necessarily fated to get the disease. She explained the oft-quoted statistic about breast cancer—a woman's risk of getting the disease is 1 in 9. "Those numbers actually refer to a woman's risk from age 20 all the way to age 80," she said. So, in actuality, "for a woman from age 20 to age 50, the risk is just 2%; from age 50 to 70, it's 6%; and from age 70 to 80, it's 3%." As she said in her book, the 11%, or 1 in 9 figure, "is obtained by adding the risk in each age category—2% plus 6% plus 3% equals 11%." Kelly told me that she saw few signs that I might carry the gene for the most strongly hereditary cancers—breast or colon cancer— because inherited cases of those cancers often occur in young people, usually before age 50. And in contrast to inherited cancers, most cases of breast and colon cancer occur after age 60. My family members had all contracted cancer in their 60s or 70s. But my family did seem to have a susceptibility to cancer, including breast, colon, skin, and pancreatic cancer. Some scientists have theorized that families like ours, in which there's a lot of cancer but no clear hereditary pattern, may have a cancer gene that hasn't been discovered yet. At the same time, my relatives' experiences with cancer did not mean that I would get the disease myself, "for cancer risk is often a combination of genetic and lifestyle factors," Kelly said. Some people in families in which there's a strong history of cancer do not get the disease at all, but the reasons are not yet known.

Then we talked about how to prevent cancer, and I confessed that my diet was far from perfect. I found it hard to eat as many vegetables as I should, and I had an unfailing sweet tooth. And to top it all off, I didn't exercise. Kelly agreed that it would be good to make some changes. "But go slowly—you don't want to make yourself feel deprived or under the gun to exercise every day," she counseled wisely.

We agreed to meet again later after I had collected my grandmother's and grandfather's death certificates. Walking out of Kelly's office, I felt relieved and unburdened.

*   *   *

I finally did take Kelly's advice—after much procrastinating—and sent away for my grandmother's and grandfather's death certificates. I also sent away for my mother's medical history at Memorial Sloan Kettering, where she had been treated. It might give Kelly more clues about my mother's cancer, she had told me.

My mother's medical records were the first documents to arrive. But, somehow, I couldn't read through them. I flipped through the pages and saw my mother referred to merely as a patient with "breast cancer metastasized to the lungs." It seemed so cold and clinical. I filed the report, still in the envelope in which it had arrived, with my files containing notes for each of my medical stories. The white envelope stood out among the morass of manila folders.

My grandfather's death record also arrived with the information I expected: death from pancreatic cancer. Then my grandmother's death record, the information that I had been eagerly anticipating but also dreading, came in the mail.

I opened the death certificate and saw that it was filled with cramped black writing in a physician's hand. It told my grandmother's story—death from pneumonia in 1941. But the surgery she had gone to the hospital for was not for breast cancer but for uterine fibroids. I couldn't quite believe it, and I had to read it over twice before it sunk in. This news meant that there was a greatly reduced chance that I had a breast cancer gene mutation. Then I noticed a page that came with the death certificate, noting that the New York City records department had a photo of my grandmother's residence on file and asking whether I would want a copy for $25? Since I thought it would make a nice gift for my father, I ordered one, and thought no more about it.

After sending the photo to my father for his birthday, I was surprised to hear from him, almost immediately after he opened the package, he said. He was a fastidiously neat man, often gruff and funny, but a man who reluctantly expressed his innermost feelings. For a time after my mother's death, he had seemed uncomfortable with his memories of her last few years. Just after her death, he had almost thrown out our family photo albums as he attempted to clean house, until my brother and I together protested loudly.

On the phone, my father's voice was filled with emotion, and I could tell he was near tears. "The picture of that house brought back so many memories for me. Thank you," he said. "It was just like I remembered it—with that white awning in front," he said.

Then he told me a story about his neighborhood in Queens, New York. His German father would send him with a nickel to the local bar for a pint of beer. "But they wouldn't let you inside if you were under 18, so you stood outside in your knickers waiting for that beer," he said.

I realized as I hung up the phone that, in my role as detective, I had gained not only knowledge about my grandmother's illness but also insight into my father's softer side. That insight would serve me well, for years later he would fight his own battle with a recurrence of lung cancer. His experience with the disease, and the friendship we forged through it, would increase my understanding of my fears about cancer. His losing battle with lung cancer—a painful cancer that spread to his spine and progressed rapidly—would show me how devastating cancer can be.

It also would inspire me to make a prevention plan for myself and add to my motivation to do the research that eventually became this book. I'd like to welcome you on a journey to gain the knowledge I gained—a journey toward learning how to accurately assess and reduce your risk for cancer. Written with my coauthor Michael Stefanek, former vice president of the Behavioral Research Center of the American Cancer Society, this book will aid you in putting in place a targeted action plan that will help you to decrease your risk of cancer and live a much healthier life.

This book is a joint effort. Most of the chapters are narrated by me; however, Dr. Stefanek provided ideas, input, and editing for these chapters. He also authored the introduction, which discusses the difference between cancer science and cancer myths; Chapter 1, which defines cancer risk; and the Conclusion, which will help those at risk for cancer to devise a game plan for the future.

Although John Wayne called cancer the "Big C," this is a disease that does not have to defeat us. The key to defeating cancer, in fact, lies in prevention, as well as early detection. By reading this book, you'll go a long way toward finding out how to take the best steps for your own cancer prevention and early detection. It's a comprehensive action plan, packed with information. I hope that this book will provide a true guidepost for helping you to devise an action strategy that will help not only to protect you against cancer but also to enable you to live a healthier and happier life.

Barbara Boughton

Acknowledgments

This has been a collaborative effort in many ways. In addition to the two authors collaborating, many experts in cancer research, advocacy, and treatment have lent their expertise in reviewing parts or entire drafts of each of our chapters and providing edits. We'd like to express our thanks to the following reviewers:

Therese Bevers, MD, Medical Director, Cancer Prevention Center, and Associate Professor, Department of Clinical Cancer Prevention, The University of Texas MD Anderson Cancer Center

Wendy Demark-Wahnefried, PhD, RD, Professor, Department of Behavioral Science, The University of Texas MD Anderson Cancer Center

Eduardo Franco, DrPH, Professor, Epidemiology and Oncology, and Director, Division of Cancer Epidemiology, McGill University Medical Center, Montreal, Canada

Sue Friedman, Founder, FORCE (Facing Our Risk of Cancer Empowered)

Stacy Gray, MD, Instructor, Hematology/Oncology, University of Pennsylvania School of Medicine, and Research Associate, Center of Excellence in Cancer Communication Research, Annenberg School for Communication, University of Pennsylvania

Marian Kerbleski, RN, CGRN, Hepatitis C Coordinator, San Francisco Veterans Affairs Medical Center

Ron Melnick, PhD, Toxicologist, National Institute of Environmental Health Sciences, National Institutes of Health

Joel Nelson, MD, Frederic. N. Schwentker Professor and Chairman, Department of Urology, University of Pittsburgh School of Medicine

Alpa Patel, PhD, Strategic Director, Cancer Prevention Study 3 (CPS-3), American Cancer Society

Rick Paules, PhD, Senior Scientist and Head, Environmental Stress and Cancer Group, National Institute of Environmental Health Sciences

Beth Peshkin, Associate Professor of Oncology and Senior Genetic Counselor, Lombardi Comprehensive Cancer Center, Georgetown University

Julia Rowland, PhD, Director, Office of Cancer Survivorship, National Cancer Institute

Debbie Saslow, PhD, Director, Breast and Gynecologic Cancer, American Cancer Society

Thomas Sellers, PhD, Executive Vice President and Associate Director, Cancer Prevention and Control Division, Moffitt Cancer Center

Michael Shelby, PhD, Director, National Toxicology Program Center, Evaluation of Risks to Human Reproduction, National Institute of Environmental Health Sciences

Kevin Stein, PhD, Director, Quality of Life Research, Behavioral Research Center, American Cancer Society

Rebecca Sutphen, MD, Director, Clinical Genetics, H. Lee Moffitt Cancer Center, Associate Professor, Departments of Interdisciplinary Oncology and Pediatrics, University of South Florida, and Director, Family Cancer Genetics Network

Frank Vitale, National Director, Pharmacy Partnership for Tobacco Cessation, University of Pittsburgh School of Pharmacy

Elizabeth Ward, PhD, Managing Director, Surveillance Research, American Cancer Society

J. Lee Westmaas, PhD, Director, Tobacco Control Research, Behavioral Research Center, American Cancer Society

Shawna Willey, MD, Director, Betty Lou Ourisman Breast Health Center, Lombardi Comprehensive Cancer Center, Georgetown University

Our thanks also to the researchers who assisted us with this book, including Leigh Boghossian, Jessica Howell, Susan Godstone, and Vanessa Leigh DeBello.

The authors also give hearty thanks to Ted Gansler, MD, of the American Cancer Society, who provided his knowledge, writing and editing skills, and much time to improving our chapter drafts. The book is immeasurably improved thanks to the work of Ted and the colleagues he enlisted to provide further needed expertise.

*   *   *

And finally, some notes of personal thanks:

I'd like to acknowledge the writers and editors who helped to make this book a reality, including Jennifer Lawler, who helped me shape the book proposal, and Noreen Henson, our editor at Demos Health, as well as my brother, Michael Boughton, and my husband, Gary Kruse, for their unwavering support and feedback during the year and a half of writing this book. And finally, I'd like to thank my coauthor, Michael Stefanek, for his considerable expertise and wisdom in helping to write, edit, and refine the book.

Barbara Boughton

I'd like to acknowledge my coauthor, Barbara Boughton, for inviting me to participate and for being so collegial during this entire process. I also would like to thank my wife, Debbie Stefanek, and daughter, Alanna Stefanek, age 11, for their patience as I added so many hours to an already busy schedule with this project. My daughter assured me that if I buy her a horse, all is forgiven. My wife is still deciding on the compensation due...

Michael Stefanek

Cancer Science or Cancer Myths: How Do You Tell the Difference?

A Professional View by Michael Stefanek

In today's Internet age, it's not unusual to find tidbits about science and health littering your e-mail inbox—giving advice about a remedy for illness or tips on maintaining wellness. Sometimes it's difficult to tell what constitutes good advice based on high-quality scientific studies, what is a reasonable suggestion based on preliminary or inconsistent studies, what is biased advice that stretches or distorts the evidence from research studies, and what is just plain bogus. This introduction will provide some tips to help you as you navigate all this information and make informed decisions about your health.

Why would anyone provide information or provide suggestions on how to prevent cancer when they are not sure the information is completely accurate?

Very often, information is based on good research, but some stories in the media take this information out of context and therefore are potentially misleading. For example, resveratrol is a substance found in red grapes, grape juice, and red wine. Moderate intake of wine has been linked to possible beneficial health effects, such as reduced risk of cardiovascular disease. However, some studies have found that high resveratrol doses can reduce cancer risk in some lab animals. Studies of resveratrol in humans are still quite preliminary. Levels of resveratrol in red wine are too low for a person drinking wine to absorb enough of this substance to achieve the doses found beneficial in animal studies. On the other hand, there is overwhelmingly clear evidence that red wine, white wine, or any other alcoholic beverage significantly increases the risk of mouth, throat, liver, and breast cancer. Nonetheless, it's not hard to find newspaper or mass media Internet headlines that imply that drinking red wine will reduce your cancer risk. Even more often, the focus of the story is that a "red wine ingredient" prevents cancer. The headline takes the information out of context to grab your attention, and the scientific details may appear only toward the end of the story, if at all.

It is true that a red wine ingredient prevented cancer (in a laboratory animal study), so the headline is not a lie. Although there are many excellent medical journalists whose goal is to provide information that helps readers to make wise health decisions, in some other publications the bar is set lower—and there is pressure to write something clever or cute that will attract and entertain readers.

Many people pass along misinformation because they believe it and are trying to be helpful. This probably accounts for most of the health tips you receive from friends and relatives. Unfortunately, many of these tips are based on information or reasoning that does not follow the scientific approach we have followed in this book. Later in this introduction I will outline some pitfalls that often lead people to make dangerous conclusions about their health. And I also will provide some tips to help you identify which suggestions are worth following and which to avoid.

Most people recognize that their relatives or neighbors or coworkers are not medical experts, and they generally apply a healthy dose of caution before following their advice. Some people tend to be more gullible when the advice comes from a celebrity. Being a talented (or at least popular) actor, artist, or athlete does not necessarily mean that someone is an expert concerning cancer or any other health issue. But many fans tend to accept the medical advice of celebrities they admire without asking themselves why. Unless you are confident that the advice is sound (and we will explain how to make this assessment), you may be risking your health.

Sadly, we feel that it is our responsibility to remind our readers that useless or even harmful health information and products are sometimes spread and sold for the wrong reasons—fame and fortune.

The quest for fame may play out on a grand scale, such as celebrities hawking an unproven remedy or their latest diet book. Or fame may be more local, such as the friend who wants to be recognized as the neighborhood expert in natural remedies and advises you to use his favorite vitamin instead of your doctor's prescription. The same applies to fortune. Unhealthy advice might be motivated by a neighbor's participation in a multilevel marketing plan to sell unproven (or disproven) products for disease prevention or treatment or, at the other extreme, by large businesses with resources for expensive advertising and lobbying (to weaken consumer protection laws and regulations).

In any industry or business, there will be a temptation to improve profits by stretching the truth or even by outright lies, and it should come as no surprise that some businesses involved in wellness and health are no exception. What may be a surprise to some is that consumer protection laws and regulations are still rather weak and that enforcement is difficult, so you still need to do some homework if you want to avoid bad health decisions.

After all, it was not until 1938 that Congress passed a law that required drug manufacturers to provide evidence of the safety of drugs marketed across state lines. That law also banned false and misleading labels on food, drugs, and medical devices. It was not until 1962 that U.S. law required any drug to be proven safe *and* effective for its stated purpose.[1]

Consumers are often surprised by the lax regulation of food product claims. For example, a recent food industry program added a "smart choices" logo with a green checkmark to some products, but there were no government standards as to what products they could choose. At one point the program included sugared breakfast cereals consisting of as much as 41% sugar by weight.[2] There are some U.S. Food and Drug Administration (FDA) regulations about health claims in food marketing, but these are complex, and it is easy to be misled by vague promises that companies are allowed to make that require little or no scientific evidence.[3]

Complementary and alternative medicine (CAM) is a diverse and frequently misunderstood category of products and practices. CAM includes complementary methods that are intended to be used together with conventional healthcare to improve health and wellness, as well as alternative methods that are generally promoted to be used instead of mainstream healthcare for the purposes of treating or preventing diseases such as cancer.[1]

Although there is some overlap between the two categories, this distinction is generally useful. Alternative methods that claim to cure or prevent cancer are in most cases either unproven or even disproven by scientific evidence but still promoted by some practitioners. Many are expensive, painful, or toxic and, when promoted for treatment, can lead patients to forego beneficial conventional treatments while their disease worsens.

Complementary methods recently have been the subject of substantial scientific research, and there has been important progress toward understanding which methods work and which don't. For example, we consider complementary methods such as meditation and yoga in Chapter 12 and review some of the growing evidence of benefit. Dietary supplements are a particularly challenging group of complementary products because their regulation does not require evidence of effectiveness in support of marketing claims, which can be misleading. For example, an herbal product can claim to support the immune system without review of any evidence by the FDA. Many people reading these claims mistakenly believe that they are supported by evidence. So, consumers may mistakenly think that these products improve the immune system in ways that reduce the severity of infections, help the immune system to prevent or fight cancer, or prevent cancers of immune system cells (such as lymphoma). We don't have enough space in this book for a thorough discussion of dietary supplements and other forms of CAM. For more information, we recommend the CAM resources at the end of this introduction.

In considering ways to reduce our cancer risk, there is no substitute for scientific evidence, although you may encounter suggestions to the contrary. Here are some tips for recognizing unscientific recommendations.

It Doesn't Rely on Science

Look for solid scientific evidence—not anecdotes. Look for results of studies that are published in respected scientific journals. Articles in these journals are not published until they have been reviewed by other experts in the field to confirm that the methods are sound and the conclusions are valid. If the only publications in support of a recommendation or product is a popular Web site, magazine, or book, then there is good reason to be suspicious. Personal stories of successful cancer prevention or treatment often can rely on emotions to persuade—and emotions can indeed be important as we make decisions. However, such stories also need to be supported by facts and evidence.

Promoters Claim It Is Too Expensive to Go Through the Testing Process

Many cancer centers now conduct scientific research on CAM using funds provided by the Office of Cancer Complementary and Alternative Medicine (OCCAM) and the National Center for Complementary and Alternative Medicine (NCCAM)—both established by the National Institutes of Health to study complementary and alternative medicine—as well as other funding sources. Typically, research proposals are presented and discussed by a group of scientists working in the area of CAM, who assess the rationale, science, and promise of the proposed new CAM approaches. OCCAM and NCCAM then can provide funding for these promising approaches. Thus, CAM approaches can indeed move forward with needed financial support so that these ideas can be tested and used for cancer prevention or treatment.

Promoters Claim It's Been Used in Traditional Healing Since Ancient Times

Some traditional remedies do work, and many of these have been incorporated into conventional/mainstream medicine. But many others do not work and appropriately have been abandoned.

I love my family, but I suspect that most of my ancestors were not much smarter than I am, and they knew even less about the scientific method. They needed to go more by guesswork and trial and error—sometimes they got it right, and sometimes they got it wrong. As Harriet Hall notes in *Skeptic Magazine* (November 2008), they got it right when they thought willow bark relieved pain—leading to the discovery of aspirin. They got it wrong when they invented trepanation, or drilling holes in the head to relieve pain.[4]

Traditional remedies sometimes seem more appealing when they come from other cultures. Traditional healers often were remarkably good at finding simple remedies for "acute" conditions that respond to treatment quickly. For example, Traditional Chinese Medicine includes herbal treatments that can improve asthma (but not as well as modern treatments). On the other hand, traditional healers did not have the research methods needed to accurately study prevention or treatment of cancer.

Promoters Claim the Treatment or Remedy Is Natural—Not Artificially Made!

For some reason, we do indeed have this bias that natural is better. But why should we expect something "natural" to be superior? After all, we are all familiar with poison ivy and strychnine, both "natural" poisons that can inflict significant damage. However, a large number of modern drugs are based on natural products from plants, molds, and so on. These sources often contain a wide variety of chemical substances. It makes sense to isolate the beneficial substances and administer them in pure form, without the other substances that may cause harmful effects.

And by so doing it is possible to standardize the dose you are taking. Yet depending on an unprocessed plant means that the dose of the active substance is unpredictable and can vary according to when it was harvested, the type of growing seasons, soil conditions, and other factors.

Sometimes natural chemicals can be improved by adding, removing, or substituting a few atoms here and there. By doing so, scientists often can strengthen the beneficial effects and reduce the side effects so that the modified or synthetic chemical is safer and more effective than the natural one.

It Worked for Me!

This is a powerful argument. Some may say that they know that they took a medicine or supplement or decreased their stress and, despite their high genetic risk of developing cancer, never developed it. Therefore, there is cause and effect. They took the product, they had a positive result, and therefore the product worked.

Yet there is a difference between "correlation" and "cause and effect." I wear my lucky hat to the game, and my team wins, so I will wear my hat every time. Most people would not really believe that their lucky hats brought the win. However, for some reason, if we take some medicine and our pain goes away (perhaps because the health problem resolved on its own or responded to some other treatment), we believe that the medicine did the trick. Maybe yes, maybe no. The medicine may just be my lucky hat. We need lots of folks wearing and not wearing their lucky hats and checking to see how their team does, or perhaps I need to wear my lucky hat under other circumstances (such as when my team is having a bad year) to see what happens before I start selling hats on eBay or renting out my lucky hat.

If a Little of Something Is Good, Then More Must Be Even Better!

This reasoning is often used in promoting extremely high doses of vitamins and minerals. Unfortunately, it's almost always false. Scientists have found that deficiency of certain vitamins and minerals is associated with higher cancer risk. So it seemed reasonable to test higher doses. Unfortunately, most of these studies have shown either no benefit or even an increased risk (for example, with vitamin A supplements and increased lung cancer risk in smokers). For more on dietary supplements, see Chapter 5.

Here Are Some More Questions to Ask Yourself, Recommended by the ACS

- Is the product "secret" and available only from a few people or seen only on television "infomercials" with claims by the author of the book that he or she has the "real" answer? Real medical knowledge is shared in journals to make effective methods more widely available.
- Are you told not to use regular medical care for cancer prevention, diagnosis, or treatment? Do the promoters attack the medical or scientific community? These are reliable signs of something that won't work.

Balancing Benefit and Risk

The field of CAM research is quite new and by its very nature is somewhat exploratory. One option as you decide on a CAM approach is to wait until there is more research. In some cases, this is wise. Another approach is to consider what is currently known about the balance of benefit, harm, and cost. There is growing evidence that some mind/body methods can improve quality of life for some people already diagnosed with cancer, especially if they have certain symptoms and side effects, for instance. Relatively little is known about whether these methods influence cancer risk. However, many are things that you do yourself (such as relaxation or meditation) at little or no cost (other than your time) and with no side effects, and they may have other health benefits (such as stress reduction). So the uncertain impact on cancer risk does not mean that you should automatically reject these methods. Some people may choose to try them, and others will prefer not to. Either choice is fine.

Get Advice From an Independent and Trustworthy Source

Ask doctors, nurses, and other healthcare professionals you trust. Ask advocacy organizations concerned about cancer in general or particular forms of cancer. Always do your research!

Ask cancer and cancer prevention experts at the National Cancer Institute (NCI) or the American Cancer Society (ACS) or oncologists (physicians who treat cancer) at your nearest National Cancer Institute Comprehensive Cancer Center. To find an NCI Comprehensive Cancer Center in your area go to https://cissecure.nci.nih.gov/factsheet/

FactsheetSearch.aspx?FSType=1.2. For information on CAM, try these respected resources:

American Cancer Society, www.cancer.org/docroot/ETO/ETO_5.asp
Complete Guide to Complementary and Alternative Cancer Therapies: The Essential Guide for You and Your Doctor, 2nd edition. Available at the ACS Web site: www.cancer.org/docroot/pub/pub_0.asp?from=fast
Office of Cancer Complementary and Alternative Medicine (OCCAM), www.cancer.gov/cam/
National Center for Complementary and Alternative Medicine (NCCAM), http://nccam.nih.gov/
Society for Integrative Oncology (SIO), www.integrativeonc.org/
Memorial Sloan-Kettering Cancer Center (MSKCC) http://www.mskcc.org/mskcc/html/11570.cfm
MD Anderson Cancer Center http://www.mdanderson.org/education-and-research/resources-for-professionals/clinical-tools-and-resources/cimer/therapies/index.html

References

1. American Cancer Society. *Complete Guide to Complementary and Alternative Cancer Therapies: The Essential Guide for You and Your Doctor*, 2nd ed. Atlanta: American Cancer Society, 2009.

2. Neuman, William. "For Your Health, Froot Loops." *New York Times*, September 4, 2009. Available at www.nytimes.com/2009/09/05/business/05smart.html

3. Hobsone, Katherine. "7 Must-Do's Before You Buy a 'Functional Food.' The Grocery Aisles Are Filled with Functional Foods That Claim to Improve Your Health. How to Choose?" *US News & World Report*, May 5, 2009. Available at http://health.usnews.com/articles/health/diet-fitness/2009/05/05/7-must-dos-before-you-buy-a-functional-food.html

4. Hall, Harriet. "Notes." *Skeptic Magazine*, November 2008.

1

What Is Cancer Risk?

A Professional View by Michael Stefanek

...In this world, nothing can be said to be certain, except death and taxes.

—Benjamin Franklin

What's in a Number?

- In 2009, about 169,000 cancer deaths in the United States were caused by tobacco use.
- Approximately one-third of the 562,340 cancer deaths in 2009 in the United States were related to obesity, physical inactivity, and nutrition.
- Up to 1 million skin cancers diagnosed in 2009 in the United States could have been prevented by protection from the sun's rays.
- Men who smoke are about 23 times more likely to develop lung cancer as compared with men who don't smoke.[1]

We are surrounded by percentages. We listen to weather reports telling us that there is a 40% chance of rain and that the humidity is 78%. As political races unfold, we try to makes sense of this and that pre-election poll and wonder if the difference between 25% and 30% really means as much as the television pundits make it sound.

I also find myself living in numbers as the parent of a 11-year-old girl. As I play a horse game with her on the computer, how do I best explain to her what a 40-to-1 long shot means (and perhaps more important, how do I console her when this long shot fades down the stretch)?

In addition to numbers in our everyday life, we are bombarded with numbers and probabilities and risk estimates for health. A drug ad claims to cut cholesterol by 40%, or we receive advice that a daily walk cuts the risk of having heart attacks by 10%.

The numbers presented in the bulleted list opening this chapter are also risk estimates, with the consolation that these numbers have the potential to change. That is, they are all related to behavior, and we can change these behaviors, providing us with the opportunity to decrease our risk of cancer. Yet how easily do you really understand these numbers and what they mean for you and your loved ones? How can you take those numbers and make them important in your life so that you and your significant others reduce the risk of developing cancer? How do you make those numbers *meaningful* to you?

Hearing the numbers is simply the first step. How we estimate our own risk for disease or risk in general is quite tricky. For instance, in 2001, the odds of dying in a pedestrian accident were 1 in 46,960, whereas the odds of dying in an earthquake were 1 in 131,890, according to the National Center for Health Statistics. Yet many people "feel" that living in an earthquake zone is riskier. Many of us are aware that it is objectively safer to fly than drive, but this does not prevent the "fear of flying" that keeps many people grounded as they buzz along at 70 miles per hour on our interstate highways.

Risk estimation is more than just numbers—it involves emotion, which may affect how people estimate their risk for cancer. Forget all the details and the mathematics underlying these estimates. What do you need to know about risk and your risk perception, and perhaps more critically, what can you do about understanding your risk?

What Should You Know?

Let's start off by getting on board with the same definition. Nothing fancy here—*risk is simply the likelihood that something will happen*. This can get a little more complicated, but we will deal with that later. Experts in medicine and health rely on numbers to help them understand risk as it applies to disease. But, as we know, risk and numbers and averages can be quite misleading.

We need only remember the joke about the man whose head was in the oven and feet in the freezer to see how numbers and averages can be misunderstood. When asked why he was doing this, the man replied "On average, I am quite comfortable." Or there's the one about the man who frantically determined the odds of a bomb being on board the plane on which he was scheduled to fly. He determined the odds, decided they were not low enough, and then carried a bomb on himself, reasoning that the probability of two bombs being on board was virtually nonexistent.

There are some numbers and figures that will be helpful for you to know for your new career as an expert in estimating your own health risk. I will keep these to a minimum, but you will see them often as you hear explanations of your risk, see ads for drugs, or read newspaper articles about cancer.

One commonly used term that you will run into is the *absolute risk*. This is risk presented as an absolute number, not as a percentage (50% reduced risk) or ratio (one-half the risk). For instance:

> Ten out of 1000 women who do not exercise regularly will develop breast cancer over the next 5 years.

Absolute risk reduction is defined as the difference in the chance that something will happen by doing or not doing something expressed in simple numbers. For instance:

> Ten out of 1000 women who *do not* exercise regularly will develop breast cancer over the next 5 years.

> Five out of 1000 women who *do* exercise regularly will develop breast cancer over the next 5 years.

Thus, the absolute risk reduction is 5 out of 1000, meaning there will be five fewer cases of breast cancer out of 1000 women due to exercise.

> For every 1000 women who exercise regularly, there will be 5 fewer cases of breast cancer.

Relative risk is simply the risk of something happening (developing cancer) if you take some action versus not taking action presented in a ratio form. For instance:

$$\frac{\text{Number of women who develop breast cancer if they exercise regularly}}{\text{Number of women who develop breast cancer if they don't exercise regularly}}$$

Let's just say, to keep things simple (more details are provided later in the book about exercise and risk), that the top number is 5 out of 1000, and the bottom number is 10 out of 1000. In this case, 5 divided by 10 is 50%. Thus an ad campaign to get people to exercise might say

> For women who exercise regularly, the chance of developing breast cancer is one-half that of women who don't exercise!

Another way of saying this—in a way that might help women to begin exercise programs—is an ad that reads

> Regular exercise reduces breast cancer risk by 50%!

In other words, this tells you the *relative* number of women saved, presented as a fraction or as a percentage—not the actual number. Thus this is the *relative risk*—how you compare *relative* to other people. In this case, the "other people" are women who do not exercise.

Now, there is one other less commonly used term that you might run into: *number needed to treat* or *number needed to screen*. Very briefly, this tells you how many people are needed for an action to be helpful or harmful. For instance, if a particular screening test saves the life of one out of every 1000 people who have the test, or if a certain drug saves the life of one out of 1000 treated patients, then the number needed to treat is 1000. This should not come up often, but I provide this so that you are "well armed" in interpreting statistics in the news, as well as in this book.

What is important to remember is that there is no "correct" way to present this information. All risk information can be given as *relative risk, absolute risk,* or *number needed to treat.* Researchers and marketers like to use relative risk because it can make small differences look large.

For instance, if a new drug A is tested against an old drug B on 1000 men, and drug A causes headaches in three of them versus one taking drug B, the relative risk of headaches with drug A may be reported as "triple the risk" in ads touting drug B. Knowing that headaches occurred in only three of the 1000 men also may be important information for you to know as you consider cost, convenience, and other factors. However, if only relative risk is provided, you may not know these exact numbers.

Gerd Gigerenzer, director of the Max Planck Institute for Human Development in Berlin and one of the leading authorities on how to determine and communicate risk, promotes the idea of *transparency*. He says that our difficulties understanding the subject of risk are not with the information itself being too complex but in *how* information is transmitted. It is too often presented in ways with which we are just not familiar. Gigerenzer is a strong advocate of presenting information clearly, cleanly, and without resorting unnecessarily to ratios, mathematics, and manipulations of numbers. Not surprisingly, he is an advocate of the *absolute numbers* approach. He gives the following example of a screening test for cancer and how the test might save lives:

- In this study, a screening test is provided to 1000 individuals, whereas 1000 individuals in the study do not receive screening.
- As these individuals are followed over 10 years, three who were screened died of the cancer that the screening test was designed to find, whereas four who were in the group not receiving screening died of this cancer.

You are trying to decide whether to spend your time and money on this screening test. The results could be presented in the following ways. Which way would make you most likely to request the test from your doctor?

1. There was a 25% risk reduction in developing cancer among people screened over a 10-year period.
2. Of 1000 people, four people in the group not receiving screening died of cancer, whereas three people in the group receiving screening died of cancer over a 10-year period.
3. If we give 1000 people this screening test, we will prevent one cancer death over a 10-year period.

If you are like most folks, before reading this chapter at least, you would be much more swayed by the 25% risk reduction. It is not that this information is inaccurate—the reduction in cancer risk from four to three is indeed 25%, but the *way* the information is presented (relative risk) makes a difference in how we react to the numbers. It also may influence our behavior.

There are some other terms that will be helpful for you to know, such as *false positive* and *false negative*. However, to keep things simple, and to avoid boring you to tears with too many definitions at one time, we will introduce these to you later in the book, during our discussion of screening tests for cancer.

So these are the basics of what you need to know to be a wiser healthcare consumer. You need to know how information is often presented and how the differences in the ways of presenting information make you *feel* and *think* about the numbers. You also need to develop a strategy on how best to get the information *you* need about *your* risk to help you make decisions to reduce that risk.

What Do I Do?

Wise consumers don't accept numbers until they understand them. They know that some numbers are more important than others, and they keep working until the numbers mean something to them. What are we trying to learn from the numbers provided to us, and what can numbers tell us so that we can do something about them?

Take the issue of which numbers are "important." Imagine that you have a coupon to use at the grocery store for 50% off one item. On this trip, you simply have to buy some milk, a few apples (notice how healthy this shopping trip is), and a huge side of beef for your relatives who refuse to read this book and insist on continuing their unhealthy eating habits. For which item might you use the coupon? Well, unless there is a major milk or apple shortage driving up the prices of these goods, you will likely use the coupon on that huge slab of fat-dripping beef. You know why, of course—the beef will be much more expensive, so saving 50% on a much more expensive item saves you much more money.

This same way of thinking applies to cancer and risk. When someone tells you that a medicine or changing your behavior results in "20% lower risk," you need to know what this "discount" means. More precisely, you need to know the answer to the question "20% lower than what?"—the price of a gallon of milk or 4 pounds of beef? If a given cancer is very common, then 20% may be very persuasive, and you may be willing to take a new medicine or change your behavior. If, on the other hand, the cancer is very uncommon, you may weigh the risks and benefits differently and arrive at a different decision. Again, there is no "right" answer. How you define a *big* or *small* risk reduction is up to you and may include weighing the side effects, inconvenience, and effort needed to achieve the reduction.

When faced with the avalanche of numbers related to health and cancer risk, what steps might we take to ensure that we really understand the numbers? And how can we make a decision that matches our values and preferences?

1. *Consider the source of the information.* If you are using the Web, is the site a reliable source of information (for example, the American Cancer Society or the National Cancer Institute)? If your healthcare provider is giving you the information, can he or she provide a source for the information—a journal article or a Web site? What does he or she think of the study on which the information is based? Are there scientists or medical groups that disagree with the results of the study or studies? If so, why?

2. *Does the information really apply to you?* Did the study or studies used to determine your risk or risk reduction include people of your sex, age, and race and individuals whose health is like yours? If not, are there reasons why your healthcare provider believes that the information still may apply to you? Does this decrease your confidence in this information at all?

3. *Make sure that you know what the risk outcome means.* For instance, if you have information on how much mammography screening for breast cancer or prostate-specific antigen (PSA) testing for prostate cancer reduces risk, what does this mean? Is this the risk for *developing* cancer? Is this the risk for *catching it earlier*? Is this the risk for *dying of cancer*? Ask your healthcare provider exactly what the numbers (however they are presented) mean—do they apply to prevention, early detection, or survival?

4. *Decide how important exact numbers are to you.* For many people, the exact numbers provided may not be crucial, and many of us may forget them over time. However, what may be important is simply to remember the "gist" of the information. That is, just knowing that you are at increased risk may prompt you to engage in more healthy behavior. At the same time, knowing that you are *not* at increased risk may help you to maintain or start healthy behaviors to keep your risk in the average or below-average range. Thus, once information is provided to you about risk in specific numbers, you may not need to keep them stored in your mind. You may just want to remember the risk "category" (low, average, high, etc.) and use this to motivate behavior change or maintenance.

5. *Ask for the information in a time frame.* There is always (or should be) a time frame associated with the risk estimate. This time frame changes with age. Very generally speaking, with lots of exceptions, cancer is a disease of aging. We are much more likely to develop cancer as we age. If you hear a risk estimate when you are 30, the 5-year risk may be much different than if you are 70, even if you take exactly the same medications and engage in the same health behaviors. Thus, when you hear your risk information, ask if this is your 5-year risk, 10-year risk, or lifetime risk (usually calculated up to age 85 or so).

6. *Ask for the numbers in absolute terms.* Although relative-risk information is helpful to researchers and statisticians, in the absence of absolute numbers, relative risk generally does not provide all the information you need. If you are told that

your risk is 50% lower if you take a given medication, ask "50% lower than what?" You may decide that you want the information in as many ways as possible. For instance, outside the health realm, if you want to learn about the defense budget, you may be satisfied to know that the 2006 defense budget was roughly $420 billion. This may be enough information for many to decide if the budget is too high or too low. However, others might want to know whether this included veterans benefits and services (it did not), how much this amounted to per American (more than $1300), and how much of an increase this was over the 2005 defense budget (roughly 5%) to make a decision about their support of this budget item.

For your decision making, you may want to know the relative risk you may have for developing or dying of cancer or by what percentage you can decrease your risk by engaging in a given behavior, taking a screening test, or starting a new medication.

7. *Appreciate that how we understand our risk usually involves more than numbers.* How we perceive our risk involves *feelings*. This may be one reason why people often fear flying more than driving. They "feel" safe owing to the control they have in driving a car, whereas the control they have when flying is in the hands of the pilot. Related to health, if your mother was diagnosed with breast cancer, had difficult treatment, and had a short survival, your interpretation of risk may be quite different from a situation in which you have no personal history of breast cancer or your mother, once diagnosed with cancer, is alive and thriving today. The exact numbers provided to you may *feel* different from the same numbers provided to others.

Although there are those who feel that we should always make decisions unfettered by our emotions and feelings, there is a growing appreciation that feelings are an important part of our decision making—and that they have a rightful place at the table. It is important to acknowledge to yourself how the numbers about your risk make you feel when you hear them and what "nonstatistical" personal experiences influence those feelings and the decisions you may make. Bad decisions can be made by relying solely on our *brain*, and bad decisions can be made by relying solely on our *heart*. Talk with family members, friends, and professionals as needed if a reasonable marriage between brain and heart cannot be found.

Another good strategy is to try "reframing" the risk. If you hear that your chances of developing cancer are 10%, does it feel the same when you flip that around, telling yourself that you have a 90% chance of not developing cancer? At times, doing so may help to lower distress, keep you focused, and not let your emotions interfere with whatever steps you hope to take to lower your risk.

You now know enough about risk to be a wiser consumer. This chapter may be a steady source of reference for you as you wind your way through Web sites, engage in conversations with your healthcare providers, and listen to the information often provided by the local and national news.

This information will not make you an expert but will provide you with enough knowledge to ask the right questions of your healthcare providers. It also will help you to interpret risk in a more comprehensive way, enabling you to make decisions about reducing your risk of developing cancer or catching it early if you do have a diagnosis of cancer.

For those very interested in this topic of risk and numeracy (how we understand or do not understand numbers), John Paulos has written a series of fascinating books on this topic, among them his first, *Innumeracy: Mathematical Illiteracy and Its Consequences* (Hill and Wang, 1988). In addition, Gerd Gigerenzer has written an excellent book for the interested lay reader, *Calculated Risks: How to Know When Numbers Deceive You* (Simon and Schuster, 2002). Another good book is *Predictably Irrational*, by Dan Ariely (Harper, 2009, the revised and expanded edition). Finally, a short but very informative guide has been authored by Lisa Schwartz, Steven Woloshin, and Gilbert Welch, all faculty members at Dartmouth College, entitled, *Know Your Chances: Understanding Health Statistics* (University of California Press, 2008).

Reference

1. American Cancer Society. *Cancer Prevention and Early Detection: Facts and Figures 2009*. Atlanta: American Cancer Society; 2009.

2

Assessing Your Cancer Risk: From the Web to Your Doctor's Office

Cancer. For those who have been touched by the disease—and that includes millions of us—worries about cancer can be a part of life. One woman with a history of cancer in her family describes it as being "the gum on the bottom of my shoes." You don't notice it until it's time to make a step forward—to get a mammogram or colonoscopy—but it's there, ever present, ready to make your life unbelievably messy.

Occasionally, as I ready myself for my shower in the morning, I catch a glimpse of the scar on my back that is left from my surgery for basal cell skin cancer. Although basal cell skin cancer is not life-threatening, just having had it makes me more at risk for melanoma—the skin cancer that may be deadly. The quarter-sized scar left on my back is a reminder of my own mortality. It's also a challenge to me to live a healthy life—to apply sunscreen every time I walk outdoors and to wear sun-protective clothing and limit my time in the sun.

In 1966, a landmark study found that 31% of a large sample of US residents said that being diagnosed with cancer was "a significant cause for worry in their lives."[1] Now we have drugs and therapies that have made it possible for many people to survive cancer for many years. Yet research has shown that many people still hold erroneous notions about this disease. A recent study highlighted the erroneous notions that many Americans hold about cancer today.[2]

- In a national survey of over 6300 adults, more than half agreed with the statement: "It seems like almost everything causes cancer."
- More than 71% agreed that "There are so many recommendations about preventing cancer; it's hard to know which ones to follow."

- And 27% agreed with the statement: "There's not much people can do to lower their chances of getting cancer."

In the study, those who had fatalistic beliefs about cancer also were less likely to put in place the very preventive health and lifestyle behaviors that would help to reduce cancer risk: exercising at least weekly, not smoking, and eating five or more servings of fruits and vegetables per day!

Holding erroneous notions about cancer can negatively impact our preventive health behaviors—making us less likely to eat a nutritious diet, exercise, give up smoking, or even get the screenings tests (such as colorectal screenings, mammograms, and Pap smears) that help to catch cancer early—and stop it in its tracks.

In another recent study, the American Cancer Society, *Prevention* magazine, and the Discovery Health channel designed and conducted a survey of 957 Americans about their beliefs on cancer.[3] The results showed that many people who took the survey could accurately identify certain misconceptions or myths about cancer. However, more than 67% of respondents believed the misconception that "the risk of dying from cancer in the United States is increasing." In fact, the risk of being diagnosed and dying from cancer has decreased since the 1990s. More than half the people diagnosed with cancer today survive the disease, and some are completely cured. Other erroneous notions spotlighted by the study included

- More than 16% of people in the study believed the pessimistic misconception that long-time smokers cannot reduce their risk for cancer by quitting smoking. In fact, after a smoker quits, and if he or she stays a nonsmoker for at least 10 years, the risk for cancers can be decreased by as much as 50%.
- Almost 40% of those questioned also believed the erroneous statement that "living in a polluted city is a greater risk for lung cancer than smoking a pack of cigarettes a day." In truth, smoking is a much bigger risk factor for cancer than is environmental pollution.

*   *   *

Fear of cancer understandably also may dog those with a personal or family history of the disease—especially if family members have died of the disease. There is nothing like a brush with cancer to give one an understanding of the destruction it can cause.

The specter of breast cancer seems to especially inspire worry among those whose family members have been affected by the disease. Studies conducted since the 1990s have found that up to 30% of women with at least one first-degree relative with a history of breast cancer have cancer-specific worries that adversely impact their daily functioning. And some groups—particularly African-American women at increased risk for breast cancer—may have strong fears about one day being diagnosed with the disease. Since the 1990s, studies of African-American women have found that 50% of African-American women with a family history of breast cancer are concerned or very concerned about their risk for the disease.[1]

Each year, when I show up at the breast clinic for my yearly mammogram, I try not to let my trepidation show. The radiology tech takes a look at me in my hospital gown and always asks the question I'm dreading, "What's your family history of breast cancer?" I feel decidedly irritable as she flattens my breast against the cold plate of the X-ray machine and pushes a glass plate down hard against the breast. "Hold your breath," she says cheerily.

The next week, at home, I get a card with the simple sentence, "We are pleased to tell you that your mammogram showed no sign of breast cancer." I am relieved and then toss the card into the garbage can so that I can quickly forget it. I am safe, at least for now.

Yet, although people like me with a personal and family history of cancer are at increased risk for the disease, the truth is that genetics or personal history *is not destiny*. There are many ways to reduce your risk for cancer and to catch the disease early—and regular mammograms, colorectal screenings, and Pap smears, as well as a host of other actions, are safeguards you can take.

Researchers now know, for instance, that lifestyle changes, such as not smoking, maintaining a healthy weight, exercising, and eating right, can cut your risk of cancer by up to 70%. So is our fear of cancer entirely misplaced? In a word, yes.

Research has found that the majority of people misperceive their risk for cancer—in most cases overestimating their risk. When my coauthor, Michael Stefanek, PhD, formerly with the American Cancer Society and the National Cancer Institute, and William Klein, associate director of the Behavioral Research Program at the National Cancer Institute, reviewed published studies about cancer risk perception in a paper published in *CA: A Cancer Journal for Clinicians* in 2007, they found that people often misinterpret information about cancer risk.[4] They tend to overestimate their own risk not because they are pessimistic but because they use statistical scales differently than do researchers, scientists, and clinicians. Statistics is a field that's not always entirely understood, even by healthcare clinicians, so it's easy to see why statistics about cancer risk can be misinterpreted by the general public.

A recent 2009 report by French researchers of over 4046 participants also found that cancer was considered to be the most serious disease—far more than HIV/AIDS and cardiovascular disease. Some of the risk factors for cancer—such as smoking, sun exposure, and alcohol use—were well known, but at the same time, many people in the study justified behaviors that increased their risk. The authors concluded that education about cancer risk is vital—to hopefully encourage all of us to take more and better steps toward prevention.[5]

What Is Cancer?

Cancer is the abnormal growth of cells. Cancer cells, unlike normal cells, grow in an uncontrolled manner and, in some cases, metastasize or spread to other parts of the body.

For those of us who want to know more about our personal cancer risk, it's important to understand the different kinds of cancer risk factors. A *risk factor* is anything that affects your chance of getting a disease such as cancer. Having one or more risk factors for cancer may mean that you could be more likely to get the disease at some point in your life compared with other people without such risk factors. And many people with one or more risk factors never develop cancers. Even if they do, it is often not possible to say which risk factors were responsible.

Some risk factors for cancer occur after you are born, and many of these can be avoided or changed—by changing lifestyle habits, such as smoking, for instance. Risk factors also include traits you are born with, such as genes inherited from your parents and your sex.

Risks That Occur During Your Lifetime

Aging is the single strongest risk factor for cancer. Although some types of cancer typically occur in children or young adults, most cancers are diagnosed in those over age 65.

Lifestyle choices, such as alcohol, tobacco use, diet and physical activity, the exposure one gets to the sun's rays, sexual behavior, and (for women) even your reproductive history, influence cancer risk. You may be surprised to learn that tobacco use, an unhealthy diet, and a lack of physical activity are the three lifestyle factors thought to most impact cancer risk today, according to the American Cancer Society.

Smoking is a huge risk factor for cancer and, in fact, accounts for one-third of all cancer deaths, including cancers of the lung, mouth, larynx, bladder, kidney, cervix, esophagus, and pancreas.

Obesity is the second most important factor leading to cancer, after tobacco. Obesity is an important risk factor for cancers as diverse as breast, colorectal, endometrial, gallbladder, pancreatic, thyroid, ovarian, cervical, liver, multiple myeloma, and even esophageal cancer. The mechanisms by which obesity lead to cancer differ depending on the type of cancer. Although fat cells are not usually thought of as "active," they in fact put out a range of hormones that include insulin-like growth factor 1, which adds to the risk of colon cancer, and estrogens, which raise the risk for breast and endometrial cancer.

Diet, including alcohol use, intake of healthy fruits and vegetables, and whether or not your diet is high in red and processed meats, also can influence cancer risk, including risk for some of the most common cancers, such as breast and colorectal cancer.

Physical activity helps to maintain a healthy weight but also independently lowers the risk for some cancers.

Hormone levels and reproductive factors, such as your age when you first start menstruating, number of pregnancies, and age at menopause, can influence breast cancer risk, as well as risk for ovarian and endometrial cancer. The exposure you get to hormones such as estrogen seems to impact your chance for breast cancer—so an earlier age at first menstruation, fewer pregnancies, and a later age at menopause all increase your exposure to estrogen and breast cancer risk.

Infections

Infections with some *viruses* or *bacteria* also increase the risk for cancer. Nearly all cervical cancers are caused by certain types of the human papillomavirus (HPV). Seventy percent of all cervical cancers are caused by two types of the HPV—types 16 and 18. Females between the ages of 9 and 26 years can reduce their risk for cervical cancer by getting a vaccine to protect them against these two HPV types. HPVs also can play a role in causing vulvar, vaginal, penile, and anal cancer.

Safe-sex habits help to limit exposure to the viruses that cause HPV, and regular Pap smears can help to catch cervical lesions before they become cancerous or find cervical cancer early when it is most treatable. (For more about preventing cervical cancer and detecting HPV, see Chapter 7.)

Other viruses, such as hepatitis B and C, increase your risk of liver cancer, and human immunodeficiency virus (HIV, the AIDS virus) also increases the risk for cancers such as lymphoma and a rare cancer known as Kaposi sarcoma. Epstein-Barr virus has been linked to an increased risk of some forms of lymphoma.

Helicobacter pylori, the bacterium that causes stomach ulcers, eventually may lead to stomach cancer and lymphoma in the stomach lining, if untreated.

The Environment

Exposure to radiation and to certain chemicals in the environment can cause cancer. *Ultraviolet radiation* from the sun, sun lamps, and tanning booths increases the risk for skin cancer, as well as causing early aging of the skin. Skin cancers are more common in southern locations, where the sun's rays are strongest. Exposure to ultraviolet radiation reflected by sand, water, snow, and ice also can increase cancer risk. Moreover, although sunlamps and tanning booths may seem more innocuous than ultraviolet radiation from the sun, there are no data to suggest that they are safer than sunlight.

Ionizing radiation is high-energy radiation that may increase risk for cancers by damaging DNA and other important chemicals of cells. This includes natural background radiation from cosmic rays, medical sources of radiation such as diagnostic X-rays or radiotherapy for cancer, and non-medical sources such as atomic bomb tests and nuclear reactor accidents. One very important ionizing radiation source is exposure to *radon*, a radioactive gas that occurs naturally in soil. Lung cancer risk can be increased by working in mines or living in homes with high radon levels. Some areas of the country also have especially high levels of radon. Home radon kits can tell you if your home has higher than normal levels of radon.

Exposure to certain chemicals and substances—such as asbestos, benzene, cadmium, and nickel—also can increase your risk for cancer. Some cancer-causing exposures, such as air pollution, affect entire communities. Others are rare in the general environment, and exposure is mostly limited to people in certain industries or occupations.

Risks That You Are Born With

A history of cancer in the family makes one more at risk for the disease. Certain types of cancer do occur more in some families than in the rest of the population—for example, melanoma and cancer of the breast, ovary, prostate, and colon. Some people inherit genetic mutations (a change in a gene that is passed from parent to child) that can increase the risk for some cancers.

However, even when the disease runs in your family, factors other than genetics may be involved in increasing your risk for cancer. Members of the same family often share the same lifestyle. For instance, my father's cigarette habit and my grandfather's regular tobacco pipe smoking increased their risk for the cancers with which they were eventually diagnosed—lung and pancreatic cancer, respectively.

Cancer is usually caused by more than one genetic mutation. One mutation may be inherited, and then risk factors later in life cause additional mutations, leading to cancer. In other words, a person may inherit a susceptibility to cancer, and then acquired factors such as lifestyle factors cause additional damage on a cellular level that eventually result in cancer. In some instances, several cases of cancer in a family may just be pure bad luck—caused by chance—according to researchers.

Race also can influence one's risk for certain cancers. Although race is a trait you are born with, this doesn't mean that differences in cancer risk related to race are due completely or even mostly to your genes. There are important racial and ethnic differences in diet, in access to healthcare, and other factors that strongly contribute to cancer disparities. Cancers of the prostate, for example, are more common in African-American men than American men of other races. But prostate cancer is also very uncommon in most of Africa.

Cancer Risk Is Complex

People have different risk factors for cancer depending on their personal history, family history, lifestyle, age, race, and even the locality where they live. At the same time, there's no need to panic. There are changes you can make that can reduce your cancer risk. You can reduce your risk for colon cancer, for instance, by 70% to 80% by not smoking, eating a healthy diet, avoiding excess alcohol intake, exercising, and avoiding excess weight gain. Getting screened for colon cancer, if you are over age 50, is also key to preventing this disease. Good weight control, a healthy diet, and substantial physical activity (more than 4 hours a week) also can reduce the risk for postmenopausal breast cancer by 30% to 35%, according to Graham Colditz, MD, DrPH, professor of surgery and medicine and associate director of the Alvin J. Siteman Cancer Center at Washington University School of Medicine.

Assessing Your Risk for Cancer on the Web

So how do you accurately assess *your* individual risk for cancer? You can start by turning to the Web.

There are several sites that now provide explanations of what cancer risk is, the factors that contribute to this risk, and self-tests that give you risk estimates for various types of cancer. These sites also provide advice on how to reduce your exposure based on your personalized risk factors for a variety of different cancers—from prostate to skin to breast cancer.

I first learned that there were Web sites where you could easily assess your cancer risk—specifically one on breast cancer risk run by the National Cancer Institute (NCI)—during my stint with a news magazine for oncologists. Since I am by nature curious, I logged on to the NCI breast cancer site. After answering seven simple questions about my reproductive, medical, and family history, I got my answer. My risk for breast cancer was above normal but not extremely high—as I had feared. I breathed a sigh of relief.

At a cancer risk assessment Web site run by the Siteman Cancer Center at the Washington University School of Medicine called "Your Disease Risk," however, I found, to my surprise, that I had a "very much above average" risk for melanoma. My blistering childhood sunburns and my family history of melanoma increased my risk, but I could lessen it by wearing sunscreen lotion every day, wearing protective clothing in the sun, seeking shade in the outdoors, and staying away from tanning booths, the site told me.

These two Web sites provided me with important information, just as they are doing for thousands of other people throughout the United States. The "Your Disease Risk" and NCI Web sites are two of the most respected and popular sources for providing information about cancer risk on the Web. In fact, the "Your Disease Risk" Web site gets 1000 visitors every day, according to its developers. There are also a number of other Web sites where you also can assess your risk of cancers, such as lung cancer, breast cancer, and gynecologic cancers.

The NCI Web site, for instance, has two interactive tools for assessing one's risk of breast cancer and melanoma. The breast cancer risk assessment tool was first developed to calculate risk for women enrolled in the Breast Cancer Prevention Trial, a large study on preventing breast cancer. At the site, a woman answers questions about her reproductive and birth history, family history of breast cancer, and personal history of breast biopsies. At the end of the test, the woman receives two numbers—one showing her risk for getting breast cancer in 5 years and the other revealing her chance of breast cancer up to age 90. These numbers are explained and compared with those for an average woman of the

These reputable Web sites provide interactive tests where you can assess your risk for cancer:

Disease Risk Index, Harvard School of Public Health
www.diseaseriskindex.harvard.edu/update/
Allows you to assess your risk of 12 different kinds of cancer.

Lung Cancer Risk Assessment, Memorial Sloan-Kettering Cancer Center
www.mskcc.org/mskcc/html/12463.cfm
Assesses the risk of lung cancer for smokers.

National Cancer Institute Risk Tools, Breast Cancer Risk Assessment Tool
www.cancer.gov/bcrisktool/
Assesses your risk for breast cancer.

Melanoma Risk Assessment Tool
www.cancer.gov/melanomarisktool/
Assesses your risk for melanoma.

Colorectal Cancer Risk Assessment Tool
www.cancer.gov/colorectalcancerrisk/
Assesses risk of colorectal cancer for men and women between age 50 and 85. At time of publication, this tool was applicable to Caucasians, African-Americans, Asian-Americans and Pacific Islanders and Hispanics/Latinos. Plans call for eventual updates to include American Indians and Alaska Natives.

National Surgical Adjuvant Breast and Bowel Project
www.breastcancerprevention.org
Calculates your risk of breast cancer.

Cancer Risk Assessment Survey Gynecologic Cancer Foundation and Women's Cancer Network
www.wcn.org/risk_assessment/
Assesses your risk of breast cancer, ovarian cancer, endometrial cancer, cervical cancer, vulvar cancer, and vaginal cancer.

Your Disease Risk, a Project of the Siteman Cancer Center at the Washington University School of Medicine
www.yourdiseaserisk.wustl.edu/
Lets you calculate your risk of 12 different kinds of cancer.

same age and with the risk of women who were involved in the Breast Cancer Prevention Trial. In this trial, the antiestrogen drug tamoxifen was evaluated against placebo in high-risk women to see if it could prevent or decrease the risk of breast cancer.

"It's valuable to have objective information about cancer risk," says Mitchell Gail, MD, PhD, the scientist who developed the statistical model that underlies the breast cancer risk assessment tool. "It puts a person's risk for breast cancer in perspective."

The NCI breast cancer risk assessment site provides a wealth of detail about the risk factors for breast cancer. It also has easily accessible information on tamoxifen and the drug's benefits and side effects. The site informs women about the current clinical trials testing preventive anticancer medications and supplements (including soy extracts), as well as results on the clinical trial called STAR (Study of Tamoxifen and Raloxifene), in which the preventive breast cancer medication tamoxifen was tested against the drug raloxifene in slightly fewer than 20,000 high-risk postmenopausal women. (For more about preventive anticancer medications, see Chapter 10.) The Web site also informs women about clinical trials on screening for breast cancer and treatments for the disease, particularly breast cancer in situ or ductal carcinoma in situ—cancer confined to the milk ducts of the breast.

The NCI Web site refers people to the Cancer Information Service, available by telephone, which provides accurate, up-to-date information on cancer. There are links to other sites that provide information about breast cancer prevention, clinical trials, cancer research, and genetic counseling and testing. At these sites you can find names and contact information for genetic counselors or clinical trials of medications and procedures designed to prevent cancer.

When I logged onto the site, I found information about the genetic counselor I chose to visit, Patricia Kelly, as well as her e-mail address. After I sent her an e-mail, I set up an appointment for genetic counseling and visited her Web site, which was filled with information about assessing breast cancer risk.

The NCI Web site also provided me with detailed information about hormone-replacement therapy (HRT) and answered some difficult questions I had about the pros and cons of HRT—a subject I had discussed with my doctors because I was nearing the age of menopause. It also provided me with a wealth of information about just what constitutes risk factors for mutations in two genes known as *BRCA1* and *BRCA2*, genes that confer an elevated risk for some familial cancers, a subject we'll discuss in more detail in Chapter 3.

What is it like to take the tests? The NCI melanoma risk assessment tool asks 11 questions for males and 10 questions for females. The questions ask where you live; your age, race, sex, and history of blistering sunburns; whether your skin is light, medium, or dark; whether you tan; and how many moles and freckles you have. Males are asked if they have ever had severe sun damage on the shoulders.

The NCI's melanoma risk assessment tool estimates an individual's risk of melanoma during the next 5-year period and up to age 70. Based on a statistical model developed during a study of 1663 non-Hispanic white patients from clinics in Philadelphia and San Francisco, this tool is designed to be used with a brief physical exam by a physician. Because the melanoma risk assessment tool has not been validated in large populations, it's best to use it only along with an exam and consultation with your physician.

The tool, in fact, is meant to be used in conjunction with a skin exam at your physician's office, says Margaret Tucker, MD, director of the human genetics program and chief of the genetic epidemiology branch at the NCI and one of the developers of the tool. "We're very excited about it. With very few questions, it captures about 90% of the risk factors for melanoma," she says.

Another Web site that provides personalized information about preventive health is the "Your Disease Risk" Web site. It has tools and tests that estimate risk for 12 different types of cancer, as well as other common diseases such as diabetes, heart disease, stroke, and osteoporosis. It is based on a review of scientific evidence on preventing cancer performed by the faculty of the Harvard School of Public Health but is now run through the Siteman Cancer Center at Washington University School of Medicine. After clicking on to the test you want to take, you'll answer a few questions about your personal history of cancer, family history, medical history, and lifestyle habits. The questions vary depending on the type of cancer in which you're interested. The breast cancer questionnaire asks about your intake of vegetables and alcohol, for instance, whereas the melanoma questionnaire asks about your sunburn history and whether or not you've taken immunosuppressive drugs. The tests take only 8 minutes.

At the end, you'll get a risk assessment from low to very much above average. Then the site provides detailed information about what you can do to decrease your risk and what you are doing right to keep your risk low. The breast cancer questionnaire, for instance, cautioned me to eat more vegetables per day but congratulated me for drinking less than one alcoholic drink per day. It then gave me seven tips for incorporating vegetables into my meals.

I also took the test for colon cancer. The questionnaire asked me if I exercised, ate red meat, had ever taken birth control pills, or had made taking a multivitamin or aspirin a daily habit. It also asked about my personal history of cancer. Since I often think of myself as having an above-average chance to develop cancer, I was surprised by the results: Compared with a typical woman my age, the test said, my risk was much below average. The reasons? I rarely ate red meat, I had taken birth control pills for 5 or more years—thought to be protective against colon cancer—and I drank less than one alcoholic drink per day. I also had changed my exercise habits recently so that I exercised for at least two and a half hours per week. Those 90-minute Saturday morning hikes around the Lafayette Reservoir with my friend Marcia were finally paying off, I thought triumphantly.

The Web site also noted that I could further reduce my risk by eating three servings of vegetables every day, taking a daily multivitamin, and, if I felt I needed it, taking a single aspirin (325 mg) four to six times per week after checking with my doctor.

I considered making the vegetable I detested, broccoli, my best friend but quickly discarded the thought. The next time I was at the grocery store, though, I picked up a bottle of multivitamins, along with my Diet Pepsi and ice cream sandwiches, as well as a handful of prepackaged vegetables. I wasn't perfect about my diet, but at least I was trying some healthy changes. I also made a mental note to ask my doctor if taking an aspirin a day would be wise, since I had a history of disease in the family. The decision of whether or not to take aspirin to prevent colon cancer should first be discussed with your doctor, the site emphasized. A discussion with your doctor would include talking about the risks and benefits of aspirin based on *your* individual risk factors and health and family history. "One of our goals is to get people to understand the message that lifestyle changes can lower your risk of cancer," says Graham Colditz, MD, DrPH, Niess-Gain Professor of Surgery, professor of medicine, and associate director of the Alvin J. Siteman Cancer Center and deputy director of the Institute for Public Health at Washington University School of Medicine, a former faculty member at Harvard, and one of the developers of the site. He also noted that one of the benefits of the site is that it provides prevention messages that are personalized for each user. The site is so popular that the developers also have introduced a Spanish version.

The cancer risk estimates on the "Your Disease Risk" Web site are based on analyses of the Harvard Nurses Health Study. The Harvard Nurses Health Study was begun in 1976 to study the long-term consequences of taking oral contraceptives. The study gradually expanded to investigate the role of diet and nutrition, as well as lifestyle factors such as obesity, exercise, and mood, on the development of chronic disease.

Cautions for Using Cancer Risk Assessment Web Sites

Experts caution that consumers who use cancer risk assessment Web sites should confer with their physicians so that they don't misunderstand the tests' results. When you don't have an opportunity to have a discussion with a healthcare professional, you may misinterpret your results. And that can be a hazard.

No risk assessment tool is 100% accurate, and none can tell with certainty whether a person will or will not get cancer. However, these tools will give you a good idea of your risk factors for cancer and how you can reduce those risks.

The sites are also not accurate for those who have previously had cancer, with the exception of nonmelanoma skin cancer. So, if you are a cancer survivor, it's best to speak with your physician or a genetic counselor to get an accurate idea of your cancer risk. If you are a survivor, your physician also can discuss the most effective ways for you to reduce your cancer risk.

These Web sites also have limitations. Some of the Web sites (such as www.breastcancerprevention.org and the NCI breast cancer risk assessment tool) use the "Gail model" for their calculations and only consider family history of cancer in first-degree relatives. Thus a woman with a strong family history of breast cancer in second-degree relatives (aunts, grandmothers, or cousins) might not get an accurate assessment of her risk from these Web sites. If you think that you have a strong family history of breast cancer or other cancers, it's wise to speak with your clinician and consider the possibility of an assessment by a genetic counselor. The "Your Disease Risk" site is also most accurate for people over age 40, according to its developers.

Other risk factors are not accounted for by the NCI breast cancer risk assessment tool. These include radiation therapy to the chest for treatment of Hodgkin lymphoma or recent migration from a country with low breast cancer rates, including rural China. The tool's risk calculation method assumes that a woman who is screened is part of the general US population.

More than 116,000 women are currently enrolled in the study. A 2008 update of the site also included risk factors highlighted in the "2008 Diet and Activity Report" from the World Cancer Research Fund and the American Institute for Cancer Research.

Across all cancers, the "Your Disease Risk" researchers estimate that their risk prediction is 63% accurate. For those that are more closely tied to lifestyle—such as lung cancer and pancreatic cancer, where risk is increased by a smoking habit—the risk estimates are even more accurate, approaching 71% to 72%.

For statistical models, this level of accuracy is actually pretty good. "With our current knowledge, we can predict risk accurately about 80% of the time. That's about as good as it gets," Colditz says.

The "Your Disease Risk" Web site also promotes legislative and community efforts to prevent cancer—such as restricting youths' access to tanning booths. It also has links to other Web sites with education information on preventing cancer.

As for me, the information I received at the Harvard and NCI Web sites convinced me that I should wear sunscreen more often and eat more vegetables and fruits. I resolved to wear that great straw sun hat I had bought in Palm Springs more often. I also made an appointment with a genetic counselor to find out more about my risk for cancer and how I could lower it.

After several nights of research on the Internet, I felt more secure in knowing how I could limit my exposure to cancer-inducing elements. The self-assessment Web sites had given me objective information about how much risk I had for cancer—as well as the opportunity to challenge and confirm my own fears. I also felt more aware and able to take action to reduce my chance of ever developing the disease again.

For me, however, this was just the start on a journey toward learning how to reduce my cancer risk. There's a lot to tell about how to reduce cancer risk and how to put together a plan to reduce your own risk—as you'll find in the following pages of this book.

Questions to Ask Your Physician About Cancer Risk

1. Are there Web sites or reading material that will help me to understand my risk for cancer?
2. Are there lifestyle changes or medications that might help me to decrease my risk or prevent cancer? If so, what changes might I make or which medications could I learn more about?
3. If my family history puts me at risk, should I consider genetic counseling or testing? Is there genetic testing for the type of cancer in my family? Where might I find out more about such testing?
4. If my family history puts me at risk, are my children and siblings also at increased risk for cancer?

5. Does my risk for cancer mean that I should get screening tests earlier or more frequently than advised for the general population?
6. If I am at increased risk, are there research projects or clinical trials of preventive strategies that I can learn more about? (Adapted from the National Cancer Institute.)

Finding Health Information on the Web

There are many helpful Web sites that can provide reputable and informative information about cancer prevention, screening, diagnosis, and treatment. The following Web sites provide comprehensive information about cancer in general and about several of the most common types of cancer:

The American Cancer Society, www.cancer.org

National Cancer Institute, www.cancer.gov

Susan G. Komen for the Cure, www.komen.org

Lung Cancer Alliance, www.alcase.org

Colon Cancer Alliance, www.ccalliance.org

While you are searching the Web for information about cancer, it's important to distinguish between factual and misleading information. Carefully consider the source of any information from the Web, and discuss it with your healthcare provider. Here are some guidelines from the NCI about what to look for in a reputable health Web site:

- Any Web site should make it easy for people to learn who is responsible for the site and its information.
- The source of the medical and health information on the site should be clearly identified.
- Health-related Web sites should give information about the medical credentials of the people who prepare or review material on the site.
- Medical facts and figures on Web sites should have references (such as articles in medical journals).
- On a health Web site, any opinions or advice should be clearly set apart from information that is based on research results.
- It's important that medical information should be current. The most recent update or review date should be clearly posted.

References

1. Hay JL, Buckley TR, Ostroff JS. The role of cancer worry in cancer screening: a theoretical and empirical review of the literature. *Psycho-oncology.* 2005;14:517–534.

2. Niederdeppe J, Gurmankin Levy A. Fatalistic beliefs about cancer prevention and three prevention behaviors. *Cancer Epidemiol Biomarkers Prev.* 2007;16:998–1003.

3. Stein K, Zhao L, Crammer C, et al. Prevalence and sociodemographic correlates of beliefs regarding cancer risks. *Cancer.* 2007;110:1139–1148.

4. Klein WM, Stefanek ME. Cancer risk elicitation and communication: lessons from the psychology of risk perception. *CA Cancer J Clin.* 2007;57:147–167.

5. Beck F, Gautier A, Guilbert P, et al. Representations and attitudes toward cancer in the French general population. *Med Sci.* 2009;25:529–533.

3

Playing Detective: Discovering Your Family History of Cancer

Many people have family members who've been diagnosed with cancer. It is, after all, a common disease. If cancer "runs in your family," you may wonder if you have inherited a genetic susceptibility. But what exactly do scientists mean when they talk about "inherited" risk for cancer? And how is a family history of cancer different from an "inherited" syndrome for cancer? The answers lie in our genes.

As early as the 1800s, scientists knew that some families were more prone to develop specific types of cancer.[1] Heredity was thought to be one factor, as were shared diet, lifestyle, or exposure to chemicals in the environment. Today, we know that cancer is a disease of abnormal gene function. Genes are segments of DNA that provide the code or instructions about how to make the proteins important for our functioning human bodies. Genes contain instructions that determine our traits, such as hair color, eye color, height, and many other characteristics. Human beings have thousands of genes that are located on 23 pair of chromosomes, which are passed from parent to child. One of each chromosome pair is inherited from your father and one from your mother.[1]

You may have heard of oncogenes, which are genes that contribute to the development of cancer, and tumor suppressors, which are genes that stop or suppress cancer growth. Some tumor-suppressor genes include the *p53* gene and *BRCA1* and *BRCA2* genes, which normally stop cancer cell growth. When you inherit a mutation—that is, a change that damages these genes—you can become susceptible to developing certain varieties of cancer.[1]

However, gene mutations that help to promote cancer may arise from other causes besides heredity, including exposure to the sun's radiation or chemical carcinogens, such as those in cigarette smoke. Aging also causes accumulation of mutations in our genes. As you grow older, you accumulate more gene mutations. This is why cancer is more common as we age. Inherited gene mutations tend to cause cancers earlier in life, as compared with cancers that are not caused by inherited mutations. Inherited mutations often cause cancer before age 50.[1]

Only 5% to 10% of cancers are the strictly inherited type. Just to be clear, though, it is not the cancer that you inherit. The genetic mutation you inherit increases your *risk* for developing cancer, sometimes to a great extent. Cancer is such a common disease that many families may have more than one member who has had the disease, especially as people age. So just because you may have several family members who have had cancer does not mean that you or your family members have inherited a genetic mutation that causes cancer. The reasons for several cases of cancer in a family may be linked to lifestyle or other risk factors, such as sun exposure or even just age—or just bad luck!

Some of the signs of an inherited genetic mutation for cancer include[2,3]

- Cancer at a young age, usually before age 50
- More than one type of cancer in the same family member
- Two or more close family members with the same type of cancer or with rare cancers
- Cancer in several generations of a family, especially if the cancers were diagnosed when the people were young
- Tumors in a gender that is usually not affected, for instance, breast cancer in men
- Bilateral tumors, or tumors on both sides of the body, for instance, cancer in both kidneys, both eyes, both ovaries, or both breasts

You can start to assess whether you have an "inherited" type of cancer by looking over this list—and thinking about whether your family history of cancer may fit. Another important step is to gather information. You may not know your entire family history of cancer—most people's knowledge of their relatives' medical histories, especially those of far-flung or deceased relatives, is incomplete. But gathering a family history can give you some clues about whether you or your family members have a genetic mutation for a familial cancer syndrome.

As you gather information, keep in mind that the stories you may have been told for years about your family's history of "cancers" may be incomplete or even erroneous. Often, to get an accurate history of your family's cancer history, you'll have to be a bit of a detective—to dig beneath the stories you may have been told for years.

Consider the story of Sue Friedman. She was diagnosed with breast cancer at age 33 and knew that her paternal grandmother had died young of "abdominal" cancer back in the 1940s. Sue's mother had died young from an aneurysm, and her father was alive and healthy. Sue never connected her own story with those of families with hereditary cancer until she stumbled on a magazine article about 8 months after her diagnosis. The article detailed the *BRCA1* and *BRCA2* breast cancer syndromes, which confer an increased risk for breast, ovarian, and other cancers, and noted that certain populations—particularly those with Ashkenazi Jewish heritage—were at particularly high risk for having the breast cancer gene mutations.

"At the time, it suddenly struck me that my paternal grandmother's 'abdominal' cancer might have been ovarian cancer," Sue says now. "My heritage is also Ashkenazi Jewish, so, when I read that article, I realized I might be at risk for hereditary breast and ovarian cancer."

Sue eventually went to see a genetic counselor and then had genetic testing. As part of the genetic counseling experience, she put together a family tree, noting all her relatives who might have had cancer, including her paternal grandmother. She was dismayed at first by how little she knew about her family's medical history and how little detail the relatives she knew were able to add. Still, Sue found the genetic counseling helpful and eventually decided to go ahead with testing. She tested positive for the *BRCA2* mutation, which confers an elevated risk for both breast and ovarian cancer.

With one child and having already had a mastectomy, Sue decided to have her ovaries removed at age 35 as a preventive step to protect against any future cancer. She also had a mastectomy on her other side, and when the breast was removed, a small amount of ductal carcinoma in situ (cancer confined to the milk ducts of the breast) was found in the second breast. She now advocates on behalf of women with high-risk breast and ovarian genetic cancer syndromes through the organization FORCE (Facing Our Risk of Cancer Empowered), which she founded. The group promotes awareness of breast and ovarian inherited cancer syndromes and education and research on genetic counseling and testing.

"It's important to me that the latest research should be available to the high-risk community," Sue says. "Unfortunately, there's a lot of misinformation out there about genetic counseling and testing. As well as helping people find genetic experts who can provide thorough counseling and testing, we promote education of both physicians and consumers about inherited cancer syndromes," she says. For information on qualifications and credentials for genetics counselors, see "How to Choose a Genetic Counselor" later in this chapter.

Like Sue Friedman, if you think you are at risk for an inherited cancer syndrome, the first place to start is by querying your relatives about your family's history of cancer. Then you can start to put together a family tree or family medical history. What are the important details to get? You should try to get medical histories, including the information provided in the following list, for siblings, children, parents, aunts, uncles, grandparents, nieces, nephews, and cousins.[4]

- Age
- Ethnicity
- Any medical conditions, including cancer, and age of onset of the condition
- The cause and age of death for relatives who are no longer living

There is now an easy-to-use Web tool that can help you complete a family medical history. It's the "Surgeon General's Health Portal Tool," an Internet-based form that you can fill out to record your family's medical history. The tool assembles your information and makes a "family tree" that you can download. However, it is entirely private, and your information is not recorded. (For more information, see the "Resources" section at the end of this chapter.)

As part of completing your family tree, you may need to request death certificates for deceased relatives. These are usually available from the health departments of the city in which your relative lived. The reason that death certificates are so important is that, in past generations, cancer often was shrouded in secrecy, and relatives may not have been told the real reason for a death. But death certificates are likely to have detailed and accurate information about your relative's illness and cause of death, including cancer.

In my own case, requesting the death certificates for both of my paternal grandparents gave me needed information. I learned that my grandmother had died in her 40s from pneumonia after undergoing an operation to remove a benign uterine fibroid, rather than breast cancer, as I had thought.

I knew, of course, that two relatives on the same side of my family—my mother and my aunt—had been diagnosed with breast cancer. During my research for my family tree, however, I also found that four of my mother's cousins had been diagnosed with breast or ovarian cancer. On my grandmother's side of the family, two of my mother's cousins—both sisters—had been diagnosed with breast cancer. On my grandfather's side of the family, one of my mother's cousins had been diagnosed with breast cancer and another with ovarian cancer. And several years ago a male cousin of my own generation had colon cancer.

Although these cancers were unfortunate, they didn't raise a red flag for a familial cancer syndrome, according to my genetic counselor. The reason was that the cancers had not occurred in close family relatives and had occurred after age 50. They were likely to have occurred because of age, not heredity.

My Aunt Mary, who had been diagnosed with breast cancer, also had tested negative for both *BRCA1* and *BRCA2* mutations. This was important information for my genetic counselor, who told me that I was most likely not at risk for a known hereditary breast cancer syndrome. So I decided not to take the genetic test for the *BRCA1* or *BRCA2* gene mutations.

Although many people know about the *BRCA1* and *BRCA2* mutations that confer an elevated risk for breast and ovarian cancer, there are many other genetic cancer syndromes. Here are a few examples of some of the most well-understood inherited cancer syndromes:

- *Hereditary breast and ovarian cancer syndromes*—Women who have mutations in the *BRCA1* or *BRCA2* gene have a 50% to 85% risk of developing breast cancer and a 15% to 40% risk of developing ovarian cancer. Mutations in the *BRCA1* gene also increase risk of cervical, uterine, pancreatic, and colon cancer. Men who have these mutations have an increased risk of developing prostate cancer. *BRCA2* mutations also increase risk for prostate, stomach, gallbladder, and bile duct cancer; melanoma; and pancreatic cancer. Genetic testing for the *BRCA1* and *BRCA2* genes are widely available.[5-7]

- *Li-Fraumeni syndrome*—Most individuals with Li-Fraumeni syndrome have inherited a mutation in the *p53* tumor-suppressor gene, and researchers suspect some other genes in the remaining cases. People with this syndrome have a higher risk of breast cancer, osteosarcoma (a bone cancer), leukemia, and tumors of the adrenal gland and central nervous system. Li-Fraumeni syndrome is very rare, but testing for it is available through cancer genetics specialists.[6]

- *Hereditary nonpolyposis colorectal cancer syndrome (HNPCC)*—People with this syndrome (sometimes called *Lynch syndrome*) have a mutation in one of four genes that monitor DNA damage in your cells. Individuals with Lynch syndrome have up to an 80% chance of being diagnosed with colorectal cancer. The mutation carries a 20% to 60% risk of endometrial cancer in women and increased risk for cancers of the brain and central nervous system, stomach, bile duct, liver, small intestine, and urinary tract. Genetic testing for HNPCC is available through cancer genetics specialists.[8]

- *Familial adenomatous polyposis*—This is caused by a mutated gene that increases the risk for colorectal cancer. People with familal adenomatous polyposis often have hundreds of polyps in the colon and rectum, and without treatment, these polyps can turn cancerous. People with familial adenomatous polyposis have an 85% to 90% chance of developing colorectal cancer by age 45. They are more likely to develop cancers of the stomach, small intestine, pancreas, thyroid, and liver, as well as some types of benign tumors.[8] Genetic testing for familial adenomatous polyposis is available through cancer genetics specialists.

- *Hereditary melanoma*—Several genes have been linked to hereditary melanoma. Mutations in the *CDKN2A* gene are associated with an increased risk for melanoma and pancreatic cancer. Mutations in the *CDK4* gene confer an increased risk for melanoma. Genetic testing is available for the *CDKN2A* gene, but it's not recommended outside research studies because scientists don't fully understand the implications of a positive test result, according to the American Society of Clinical Oncology. Genetic testing for the *CDK4* gene is not yet available.[9]

- *Hereditary pancreatic cancer*—A number of genetic syndromes are associated with an increased risk of pancreatic cancer. In addition to the *CDKN2A* mutations that also cause hereditary melanoma, an inherited tendency to develop pancreatic cancer can result from hereditary pancreatitis, which involves inflammation and swelling of the pancreas. Pancreatic cancer is also more common among people with Peutz-Jeghers syndrome, a disorder that also causes many polyps in the digestive tract. Testing for these syndromes is available through cancer genetics specialists.[10]

- *Hereditary medullary thyroid cancer*—Inherited mutations in the *RET* gene can cause medullary thyroid cancer, which is a type of thyroid cancer that occurs in 5% to 10% of thyroid cancer patients. In some families these mutations only cause familial medullary thyroid cancer (FMTC), but in others they also lead to syndromes that include tumors of other glands—multiple endocrine neoplasia (MEN) types 2A and 2B. Testing for these rare syndromes is available through cancer genetics specialists.[11]

- *Hereditary kidney cancer*—Several syndromes confer an increased risk of kidney cancer. One of these is the Von Hippel–Lindau (VHL) syndrome, which confers a 40% risk of kidney cancer, as well as an increased risk for benign tumors or cancers of the eye and ear, brain and spinal cord, and adrenal glands. Other syndromes associated with kidney cancers— hereditary non-VHL syndrome, clear cell renal cell carcinoma, and hereditary papillary renal cell carcinoma—increase the risk of certain types of kidney cancers or multiple kidney tumors. Testing for some of these syndromes is available through cancer genetics specialists.[12]

Genetic Testing

Genetic testing involves taking a blood or tissue sample to test for a genetic mutation that confers an elevated risk for cancer. Unless you have already been diagnosed with cancer, guidelines recommend that you should only consider genetic testing if you are aware of a strong family history of cancer. A genetic test does not screen for cancer. That is, it is not like a mammogram or colonoscopy, which might tell you whether or not you have cancer at the time of testing. However, genetic testing along with counseling can provide a wealth of information about one's risk for cancer. If you're considering genetic testing, it's important to have counseling beforehand—to make sure that you want to go through a test and to discuss in advance your options for managing cancer risk. Counseling also will help you to prepare for some of the emotions that may occur after going through such an important experience as a genetic test for cancer. Genetic counseling also can be crucial after you receive your test results—a counselor can interpret and help you to understand the test results and suggest ways to communicate the results to your family. Whether your test result is positive or negative, you may have some emotions about it, and a genetic counselor can help you to deal with these feelings. He or she also can make sure that you get quick and appropriate follow-up from medical clinicians—clinicians who can help you to plan the next steps for your healthcare. If you go through a genetic test for cancer and test positive, your clinician may advise you to go through more screenings for cancer than the average person or may advise that you institute preventive strategies—such as taking preventive medication or undergoing a prophylactic operation. If you test negative for a genetic mutation for a familial cancer syndrome, even if the mutation has been found in your family, you still have at least the average risk for developing cancer and should undergo screening tests recommended for the general population. If there is a strong family history of cancer, however, but a mutation has not been found in your family members with cancer, you and your family still may be considered at high risk for cancer.

Going through genetic testing can be an emotional experience—no matter the outcome. In 2000, Janice Page had genetic testing for the *BRCA2* gene mutation, which runs in her family, and heard the news that she did not have the mutation. The results made her feel newly hopeful about her life, she says. "I have pretty much assumed I would always get breast cancer," she wrote in a *New York Times* article about her experience. Her older sister Patty died in 1984 after a 2-year battle with the disease, and at age 54 her sister Nancy was told she had stage III ovarian cancer. Her sister Carol, who was 53 at the time, decided to get tested and turned out to have the *BRCA2* mutation. She had her ovaries and uterus removed, scheduled mammograms twice a year, and began taking the drug tamoxifen to help prevent breast cancer.

Janice, meanwhile, at age 39, was struggling with the question of whether or not to have children because offspring of those with a mutation have a 50% chance of inheriting the mutated gene. When she heard that her test results were negative, she was stunned, she said. "I had been prepared for bad news. This was a novelty. Now I had no excuse to delay living a normal life, as a person without reason to ponder her genetic fate," she wrote in the *New York Times* article. "I felt almost a duty to go out and multiply." After attempting to have a biologic child with her husband, Janice adopted a daughter, Zoe, who is now age 5. "I really wanted to have information about whether I had inherited the mutation," says Janice, now 46 and a writer and *Boston Globe* editor. "If I had information—then I could take action, perhaps have screening tests more often, or take preventive medication."

Just as genetic testing had its positive sides—it gave her information and relief from anxiety—it also had its drawbacks, Janice discovered. After receiving her test result, "A disturbing sense of separation settled in," she says. "I had always shared everything with my sisters. Now they belonged to a club that I didn't necessarily want to join but still hated being shut out of," she said. "I wondered guiltily why I was the lucky one. . . . Having the test definitely lifted a burden—but I also felt survivors' guilt," she says. Research suggests that these feelings of guilt are not unusual. Test results of family members often can highly affect people's feelings of distress after receiving their own genetic test results for cancer. This is why genetic counseling is so vital—it can prepare one for the varying emotions that can accompany hearing test results, which may include distress, anxiety, and depression.[13]

The three most common mutations that can cause genetic cancer—the *BRCA1* and *BRCA2* gene mutations for breast cancer and the *HNPCC* gene mutation—may carry as much as an 80% risk of someday getting the cancer. With statistics like these, it's not uncommon for people at higher-than-normal risk for these cancers to experience qualms about undergoing genetic testing. Yet those who fear a positive test result may be underestimating their ability to cope. It seems that human beings are remarkably resilient. Most people who undergo genetic testing, even those who receive positive test results, are not subject to high levels of depression or anxiety, according to scientists interviewed for this book.

Research has revealed that only a minority of subjects undergoing tests for hereditary cancer experiences serious depression or anxiety. People who receive a negative test result often have a reduction in anxiety, according to scientists interviewed for this book. And surprisingly, a positive test result does not usually result in increased depression. "A positive test result often motivates people to put a healthcare plan into action—a plan that works for them individually," says Kathryn Kash, PhD, associate professor in the departments of health policy and psychiatry and human behavior at Thomas Jefferson University in Philadelphia.

Making a healthcare action plan was crucial for one family diagnosed with familial medullary thyroid cancer syndrome. After Robert (not his real name) learned that both his father and sister had been diagnosed with medullary thyroid cancer, he decided that he should be tested for the presence of the same disease. As it turned out, he also had the cancer—and so did his two other sisters. All were treated by having their thyroid glands removed and were put on medication to supply thyroid hormones. Because of their very strong cancer history, the family was diagnosed with familial medullary thyroid cancer, even though they tested negative for the gene mutation that is usually found in this syndrome. About 15% of those with familial medullary thyroid cancer test negative for this mutation.[14]

Because of their extremely strong cancer history, the family decided to work with researchers at Stanford University and Ohio State University to find out more about their inherited syndrome, and they underwent a linkage analysis—a genetic analysis in which scientists search for possible mutated genes that may be a cause of a familial disease. As it turned out, the researchers did find a mutated gene that all family members had in common and developed a genetic test for it. Then Robert's daughters, now age 7 and 11, could be tested for the genetic mutation. Results revealed that his younger daughter had the mutation—although his older daughter did not. So, at age 6, his youngest daughter had preventive surgery to remove her thyroid at the University of California–San Francisco, and cancerous cells were found in her thyroid tissue.

"I really wanted to protect my children—and I'm very glad that we had the surgery as soon as we did, because it prevented her from having to go through cancer," Robert says. Now on thyroid medication, his younger daughter has experienced no health problems. "What we did as a family was to try to educate ourselves as much as possible and make the best choices for our children," he says.

Going through genetic testing is often a decision that has to be made individually—after considering all the pros and cons. In the past, many people hesitated to go through genetic testing because of fears about insurance or employment discrimination. However, passage of the Genetic Information Nondiscrimination Act in 2008 made such discrimination illegal. The law protects those who have a genetic susceptibility to a disease from discrimination by health insurers and employers; however, it does not cover life, disability, or long-term care insurance. Tests for gene mutations that confer an elevated risk for cancer are protected under the Genetic Information Nondiscrimination Act, including the tests for the *BRCA1* and *BRCA2* gene mutations and the *HNPCC* gene mutation. However, despite such legal protections, people who undergo genetic testing and receive a positive test result sometimes still fear job discrimination for themselves and their relatives.

One example is Lauren (not her real name). At first, she didn't connect her personal and family history of cancer with a genetic mutation. Diagnosed at age 46 with colon cancer that had metastasized to her liver, Lauren had a series of treatments, including surgery, chemotherapy, and other anticancer drugs. However, when her two sisters—who both had experienced breast cancer—became concerned about the history of breast cancer on the maternal side of the family, Lauren also began wondering if she might have a genetic syndrome that put her at risk for colon and other cancers.

On her father's side of the family, Lauren's grandmother had died of colon cancer, and her uncle had experienced the disease in his 50s. Two of her brothers also had experienced cancer—one cancer of the stomach and the other cancer of the bile duct. As it turned out, Lauren's sisters were tested for the two genetic breast cancer syndromes, *BRCA1* and *BRCA2*, but their tests were negative. Lauren's test for the genetic syndrome known as Lynch syndrome or HNPCC, however, came back positive.

"My first thought was, 'What does this mean for my children?'" Lauren said. "And 'What does this mean for my brothers and sisters, and for my uncle's children?'" Out of eight siblings, Lauren's two brothers and a sister also tested positive for Lynch syndrome. Several of her nieces and nephews also tested positive. Luckily, her two sons, ages 20 and 21, tested negative.

"I felt that the knowledge I gained by taking the test was very powerful," Lauren said. After testing positive, Lauren decided to adopt a strategy of increased surveillance and has regular medical tests for the cancers for which she is at risk, including colorectal, endometrial, ovarian, and stomach cancer. Now cancer-free, she is on disability from the company where she works and has health insurance. Yet Lauren is concerned about the effects the genetic test results will have on her nieces' and nephews' chances for employment. "I know there are laws out there to protect us, but I still worry about it," she says.

As a result of her experience with Lynch syndrome, Lauren has become convinced of the importance of knowing your family's health history, including family history of cancer. "It's important to be proactive and have knowledge about your ancestors' and relatives' health history," she said.

People should be counseled extensively before and after undergoing genetic testing to ensure that they are making truly informed decisions about genetic testing, to reduce the incidence of depression and anxiety afterward, and to improve communication about cancer risk among families, geneticists say. And, in fact, many people who go through genetic testing do get such counseling because most of the testing is done in large academic medical centers.

Those who receive positive test results also should be made fully aware of their options—including the benefits and limitations of surgical and other medical preventive steps, genetics experts say. Researchers agree that people who have a family history of cancer should be getting good counseling about the risks of genetic testing and how to make choices about preventive strategies.[15]

New Developments in Genetic Testing

In the past 5 years, as the human genome has been decoded, there's also been a rapid expansion of the availability of a new phenomenon—direct-to-consumer genetic testing that is marketed and available for purchase online. Genetic testing is promoted online for everything from diabetes to cancer susceptibility, including the *BRCA1* and *BRCA2* gene mutations. Several companies are also offering and marketing even newer genetic tests. These tests search for single-nucleotide polymorphisms (SNPs) that may confer an above-average risk for certain diseases, including cancer.

Yet many genetics experts affiliated with universities say that these newer tests have not yet been proven useful in the general population. How valid the tests are in terms of predicting risk or how useful they are in helping patients to plan their healthcare is an open question. These tests are so new that no one knows for sure whether any preventive health strategies will have an effect on a person's risk profile, for instance. "What we have is early market entry of these tests before there's an appropriate amount of clinical data to show the tests' utility," says Stacy Gray, MD, instructor at the University of Pennsylvania School of Medicine and hematology/oncology and research associate at the Center of Excellence in Cancer Communication Research at the Annenberg School for Communication of the University of Pennsylvania. "These tests hold promise for the future, but we're not able to use them on an individual basis to help a patient make healthcare decisions," she adds.

The new tests look for certain SNPs—tiny differences scattered across our 23 pair of chromosomes. A strand of DNA is made up of units called *bases*, and each strand of DNA has about 3 billion bases. Within about every 1000 bases, every human being will have an identifiable "difference," or SNP. Most SNPs do not cause disease, but recent research has tied some SNPs with an increased susceptibility for certain diseases, including diabetes, heart disease, and breast and prostate cancer.

The availability of this testing has stirred controversy. Many experts fear that the easy availability of genetic testing that can be purchased via the Internet can lead to misinformation and, in the worst-case scenario, erroneous test results. Because there's no federal regulation of these companies, the labs they use may not have the quality review or standards that would guarantee the accuracy of their tests. Some also question the clinical utility of tests that online genetic testing companies say are "cutting edge," such as those that test for cancer susceptibility using SNP markers.

The tests can be obtained simply by filling out an online form and sending in a swab sample taken from inside one's cheek, a saliva sample, or by getting a blood test. Some online testing companies provide instructions or a doctor's order that one can take to a nearby lab for blood tests, such as those necessary for testing for the *BRCA1* and *BRCA2* gene mutations. Consumers usually get a detailed explanation of their test results in writing or via a personalized and password-protected Web site and can request genetic counseling over the phone. Some genetic testing companies provide counseling as part of their fees, which range from several hundred to several thousand dollars.

Genetics Experts Oppose Direct-to-Consumer Genetic Testing

Many genetics experts caution against genetic testing that is marketed online. One concern is that many genetic tests don't provide an accurate, or telling, picture of cancer risk. Rebecca Sutphen, MD, director of clinical genetics at the H. Lee Moffitt Cancer Center and Research Institute in Tampa, Florida, explains that many of the new SNPs associated with cancer increase the risk for the disease by only 50% compared with the general population. Although this may sound like a big increase in risk, it's actually not. For instance, if someone in the general population has a 10% risk of getting a disease, even a 100% increase in risk is only a 20% chance. Think of these percentages as one would gambling odds. A 20% chance of something happening—whether it's a disease or a roll of the dice—is fairly unlikely. "In the future, we might have the capability to assess several genetic changes associated with a type of cancer, but any of these may have only a small effect on your risk," Sutphen adds.

Others are concerned because online genetic testing companies are not held to the same regulatory standards of confidentiality as are hospitals and clinicians in practice. "There's also a huge spectrum of tests available, and it's difficult to judge the quality of the tests from these companies' Web sites. The problem is that the information most consumers read on these Web sites is advertising—promotion for their testing services," Gray says.

Experts are also concerned that direct-to-consumer genetic testing may create unnecessary worry among those who test positive for cancer susceptibility based on SNP testing. Others who test negative may feel falsely reassured, and negative test results may lead some consumers to neglect screenings and healthy lifestyle choices. Without the follow-through that genetic counseling provides, such testing may create more questions than answers for consumers.

It all adds up to a scenario in which consumers may not be getting the information they need about the genetic tests being offered by online companies. "Direct-to-consumer genetic testing is a huge problem because there's no guarantee of genetic counseling. And without this counseling, you don't know what to do with a test result—what it means for future healthcare decisions," Kash says.

Many experts doubt that online companies can provide sufficiently thorough counseling and follow-up—which many people going through genetic testing often need. "Sometimes the test results (for instance, for the *BRCA1* and *BRCA2* genes) are not black and white. For *BRCA1* and *BRCA2* gene testing, one can get an 'inconclusive' result," says Nicki Chun, MS, genetic counseling supervisor at the Stanford Medical Center Genetics Clinic. "I would be afraid that people who get an 'inconclusive test' result would not get the counseling and follow-up they need for making decisions about their healthcare," Chun says. "Ideally, everyone going through genetic counseling and testing should get a proactive roadmap that they can follow to make decisions about their healthcare—now and in the future."

Research shows that whether one gets a negative or positive test result from a genetic test for a cancer syndrome such as *BRCA1* or *BRCA2*, it's likely that one will need ongoing support. Genetic counseling can help one to make healthcare decisions over time, provide emotional support as one deals with the health implications of a test result, and assist in communicating with family members about the genetic testing process and test results. And online testing companies are simply not able to offer such extensive and wide-ranging support, many experts argue.

"Most healthcare experts see direct-to-consumer genetic testing without expert genetic counseling as a risky situation," Sutphen says. "Undergoing genetic testing such as that for the *BRCA1* and *BRCA2* gene mutations is an important decision with a lot of ramifications. A positive test result could mean surgery to remove one's breasts and ovaries. So genetic counseling is quite important."

At the same time, genetic counseling is still not widely available—for instance, in rural areas of the United States. Yet new companies are stepping in to fill this need. Sutphen is on the board of a company founded by a board-certified genetic counselor called Informed Medical Decisions, Inc., that provides genetic counseling by board-certified specialists available over the telephone. Aetna has already contracted with Informed Medical Decisions to provide this service nationwide for its members who are interested in considering genetic testing. Sutphen notes that phone consultations are one way to improve access to genetic counseling throughout the United States.

Indeed, I went through part of my genetic counseling by telephone, and I found the process to be both thorough and informative. It answered my questions about my possible risk for the *BRCA1* and *BRCA2* gene mutations and reassured me that I was not at risk for a familial cancer syndrome.

I also took a thorough look at several direct-to-consumer genetic testing Web sites and considered the possibility of undergoing genetic testing for several newly discovered SNPs that might confer an increased risk for cancer. The tests might tell me if I had a genetic marker that could increase my susceptibility for breast, colon, or prostate cancer—but only if I forked over at least several hundred dollars.

However, I already felt pretty informed about my risk factors for cancer—and had made a plan to decrease those risks. In the end, I felt that paying several hundred dollars would leave me poorer but not more well informed because most of the experts I had interviewed consider the tests unproven. Instead, I decided to put my faith in making some definite lifestyle changes—lifestyle changes that can truly impact cancer risk, as you'll find in the following pages.

Do You Need Genetic Testing for a Cancer Syndrome?

Here are the steps to take to find out:

- Talk with your relatives to find out your family history of cancer.
- For relatives who have died, ask other relatives about the cause of death and age of death.
- Request death certificates from the health department of the city in which your relative lived, died, or both.
- Request a referral to genetic counseling for cancer from your physician. Ask to be referred to a board-certified genetic counselor.
- To find genetic counselors, try the directory at this National Cancer Institute Web site (www.cancer.gov/search/geneticsservices/).

How to Choose a Genetic Counselor or Specialist

Many professionals provide genetic counseling—but how do you tell who is most qualified to advise you? According to the National Cancer Institute, cancer genetics counselors or specialists should be licensed, certified, or eligible for board certification in their profession—whether that be oncology, nursing, psychology, social work, or clinical genetics. They also should be affiliated with an interdisciplinary medical team with substantial experience in cancer genetics and have advanced training or professional experience in cancer genetics. This experience could include authorship of scientific publications on genetics, courses in clinical genetics, or being a researcher on genetics clinical trials. Other credentials that can indicate a genetic counselor's expertise may include affiliation with

- American College of Medical Genetics
- American Society of Clinical Oncology
- American Association for Cancer Research
- American Society of Human Genetics

- International Society of Nurses in Genetics
- National Society of Genetic Counselors
- National Society of Genetic Counselors Special Interest Group in Cancer
- Oncology Nursing Society
- Oncology Nursing Society Cancer Genetics Special Interest Group[16]

Resources

The "Cancer Genetics Page" of the National Cancer Institute Web site: www.cancer.gov/cancertopics/prevention-genetics-causes/genetics.

For information on genetic testing and counseling, the American Cancer Society: www.cancer.org/docroot/MBC/content/MBC_2_3x_Genetic_ Testing_and_Counseling.asp?sitearea=MBC.

For information about hereditary cancer in women and the *BRCA* mutations, check out the FORCE (Facing Our Risk of Cancer Empowered) Web site: www.facingourrisk.org/.

The Surgeon General's Family Health Portrait Tool; available at https:// familyhistory.hhs.gov/fhh-web/home.action.

References

1. American Cancer Society. *Heredity and Cancer*. Available at www.cancer.org/ docroot/CRI/content/CRI_2_6x_Heredity_and_Cancer.asp?sitearea=&level=. Accessed July 15, 2009.

2. American Cancer Society. *Genetic Testing: What You Need to Know*. Available at www.cancer.org/docroot/PED/content/PED_11_3X_Genetic_Testing.as p?sitearea=PED&viewmode=print&. Accessed July 15, 2009.

3. National Cancer Institute. *Cancer Genetics Overview*. Health Professional Version. Available at www.cancer.gov/cancertopics/pdq/genetics/overview/ healthprofessional. Accessed July 15, 2009.

4. American Medical Association. *Family Medical History in Disease Prevention*. Chicago: AMA; 2004

5. National Cancer Institute. *BRCA1 and BRCA2: Cancer Risk and Genetic Testing*. Available at www.cancer.gov/cancertopics/factsheet/risk/brca. Accessed July 15, 2009.

6. American Society of Clinical Oncology. *Cancer.net: The Genetics of Breast Cancer*. Available at www.cancer.net/patient/Learning+About+Cancer/Genet- ics/The+Genetics+of+Breast+Cancer. Accessed July 15, 2009.

7. American Society of Clinical Oncology. *The Genetics of Prostate Cancer.* Available at www.cancer.net/patient/Learning+About+Cancer/Genetics/The+Genetics+of+Prostate+Cancer. Accessed July 15, 2009.

8. American Society of Clinical Oncology. *Cancer.net: The Genetics of Colorectal Cancer.* Available at www.cancer.net/patient/Learning+About+Cancer/Genetics/The+Genetics+of+Colorectal+Cancer. Accessed July 15, 2009.

9. American Society of Clinical Oncology. *Cancer.net: The Genetics of Melanoma.* Available at www.cancer.net/patient/Learning+About+Cancer/Genetics/The+Genetics+of+Melanoma. Accessed July 15, 2009.

10. American Society of Clinical Oncology. *The Genetics of Pancreatic Cancer.* Available at www.cancer.net/patient/Learning+About+Cancer/Genetics/The+Genetics+of+Pancreatic+Cancer. Accessed July 15, 2009.

11. American Society of Clinical Oncology. *The Genetics of Thyroid Cancer.* Available at www.cancer.net/patient/Learning+About+Cancer/Genetics/The+Genetics+of+Thyroid+Cancer. Accessed July 15, 2009.

12. American Society of Clinical Oncology. *Cancer.net: The Genetics of Kidney Cancer.* Available at www.cancer.net/patient/Learning+About+Cancer/Genetics/The+Genetics+of+Kidney+Cancer. Accessed July 15, 2009.

13. Vadaparampil ST, Ropka M, Stefanek ME. Measurement of psychological factors associated with genetic testing for hereditary breast, ovarian and colon cancers. *Familial Cancer.* 2005;4:195–206.

14. National Cancer Institute. *Genetics of Medullary Thyroid Cancer.* Health Professional Version. Available at www.cancer.gov/cancertopics/pdq/genetics/medullarythyroid/healthprofessional. Accessed July 15, 2009.

15. Boughton B. Genetic testing intensifies research on psychological impact of cancer. *J Natl Cancer Institute.* 2000;92:1711–1712

16. National Cancer Institute. *Cancer Genetics Services Directory.* Available at www.cancer.gov/search/geneticsservices/Accessed July 15, 2009

4

Protect Yourself Against Skin Cancer

Skin cancer is a serious health problem around the world, and it's considered epidemic today. It's the most common form of cancer in the United States, and its incidence has increased dramatically over the past few decades. One in five Americans will be diagnosed with skin cancer during their life, and one American dies every hour from melanoma, the lethal form of skin cancer, according to the Skin Cancer Foundation.[1] The American Cancer Society estimates that there will be more than 1 million new cases of nonmelanoma skin cancer and 68,720 new cases of melanoma in 2009.[2,3] The reasons for this epidemic of skin cancer? Overexposure to the sun, failure to take "sun safe" precautions, and exposure to tanning beds are three contributing factors. Although alabaster skin was once considered a mark of the upper class, since the end of World War II, tanned skin tragically has been promoted as a symbol of attractiveness, wealth, and health—a sign that one can afford vacations in tropical climates. "People like Coco Chanel, who tanned on the Riviera, popularized the idea that a tan was attractive. Thus, after World War II, vast numbers of people got extensive amounts of sun," says Clay Cockerell, MD, professor of dermatology and pathology at the University of Texas Southwestern Medical Center in Dallas. "Prior to World War II, sun exposure was considered more negative."

Nearly 30 million people in the United States also tan indoors, and 2.3 million of them are teenagers, according to the Skin Cancer Foundation.[1] And many teens expose themselves to artificial and natural ultraviolent radiation with increasing frequency as they grow older and into adulthood—even though they're aware that these practices are unsafe.[4]

The consequences for this unsafe ultraviolent radiation exposure can be considerable. It's thought to be one factor that contributes to melanoma skin cancers. The incidence of melanoma increased sharply by 6% per year during the 1970s and then by about 3% per year during the 1990s, but it has been stable since 2000, according to the American Cancer Society.[5] The American Cancer Society estimates that there will be 8650 deaths from melanoma in 2009.[3]

Basal cell carcinoma (BCC) and squamous cell carcinoma (SCC) are skin cancers that are far more common than melanoma. Most, but not all, of these forms of skin cancer are highly curable. However, left untreated, they can spread and cause disfigurement and sometimes even serious health problems.

That's the bad news. The good news is that many skin cancers are preventable, and taking some "sun safety" health steps can reduce your chances of getting this disease. But it's not as simple as just patting on sunscreen when you go for a long hike in the sun or spend a day at the beach. Reducing your risk for skin cancer requires using a variety of methods to prevent overexposure to the sun.

Know Your Skin

The skin is one of our most precious organs. I was reminded of this one day at the beauty salon when the young woman rinsing out my hair gave me a gentle compliment. "You have beautiful skin," she said. Because I have undergone surgery for BCC, that compliment reminded me of what a gift our skin is. The skin is actually the largest organ in the body. It covers the internal organs and protects them from injury, serves as a barrier to germs, and prevents the loss of too much water and other fluids.

Although the skin can seem simple, it is in fact a multilayered wonder. It has three layers: the epidermis, the dermis, and the subcutis. The top layer is the epidermis—and it's thin—about 1/100 of an inch thick. The epidermis protects the deeper layers of the skin and the organs of the body from the environment.[5,6]

Since it is the layer that is most exposed to the sun, the epidermis is where most skin cancers begin. Melanoma starts in cells called *melanocytes*, cells that make the brown pigment called *melanin*. It is melanin that makes us tan. Groups of melanocytes can form in clusters called *moles*, which can be flesh-colored, pink, tan, or brown and usually are smaller than a pencil eraser. Think of moles as benign growths. They're not cancer, and they don't spread to other parts of the body. However, when damage occurs to the melanocytes, they can become malignant or grow uncontrollably. Frequently, the first sign of a melanoma is a mole that has changed in color, size, or shape.[7]

SCCs are named for the cells in which they arise. The squamous cells make up most of the upper layer of the skin, the epidermis. BCCs arise in the basal cells, which line the deepest layer of the epidermis.[8]

BCCs are usually slow-growing, and this cancer is fairly easy to treat when detected early. Although they are rarely life-threatening, if BCCs are left untreated, they can invade the skin around them and sometimes bone and cartilage. Most people who get skin cancer will have BCC. SCCs, like BCCs, usually develop in sun-exposed areas such as the face, neck, ear, lip, and hands. They tend to be more aggressive than BCCs and can spread to fatty tissues underneath the skin. SCCs also can metastasize, or spread, to other parts of the body, although this is uncommon.[6] When a dermatologist cut off the BCC from my back, it all seemed deceptively easy. I even returned to work that same day. However, as the years went by, I learned what that BCC really could mean. In researching my work for oncology magazines, I learned that having had one BCC increased my risk for another kind of skin cancer (including melanoma) later on in my life or for developing new BCCs elsewhere on my skin. Because I had a history of childhood sunburns and my mother had been diagnosed with melanoma, I also was at increased risk for melanoma. And melanoma is a skin cancer that can spread rapidly and kill quickly, if not caught early.

So I learned to be careful about going out in the sun. Years ago, I also started applying a makeup containing a sunscreen with a skin protection factor (SPF) of 15 to my face every single day. I also became a connoisseur of hats. Trying to find hats that were beautiful and provided sun safety became my annual challenge. I finally found two hats that met my criteria for sun safety and attractiveness. One was a tightly woven wide-brim straw hat, and another was a light green cotton "shade hat" with a decorative ribbon in the front (and several inches of fabric that cascaded downward, covering my neck). Both shielded my face and neck from the sun and were easy to pack on a recent trip to Peru! To find out more about recommended types of sunscreens and hats, see the "Rules for Sun Protection" and "What Does SPF Mean?" found on pages 50–51.

Who is most at risk for skin cancer? Fair-skinned people who sunburn easily are most at risk, but skin cancer can happen to anyone. Excessive exposure to the sun's ultraviolet (UV) light is one of the most important risk factors for melanomas and other skin cancers. However, melanoma can occur (uncommonly) on parts of the body that are not exposed to the sun, although researchers don't entirely know why.

Fair-skinned people who are "weekend tanners"—that is, they're exposed to intense bursts of sunlight for short periods—are also more likely to get skin cancer, including melanoma, according to some studies.[9,10] Melanoma also can run in families, and those with a strong family history of melanoma are at increased risk.

In addition to family history, and our fair-skinned and "weekend tanner" friends, other factors that can add to one's risk of nonmelanoma skin cancer and melanoma include

- Previous bouts of melanoma or other skin cancers
- Having skin with lots of moles and freckles
- Having fair skin that sunburns easily
- Exposure over many years to UV light, either outdoors or in tanning salons
- Living in sunbelts or sunny parts of the world
- Having a weakened immune system. People who have weakened immune systems are more at risk than the average person for skin cancer. This group includes people with lymphoma and HIV infection and those having been treated long term with medications used to prevent organ rejection after an organ transplant.[5,6-8]

Clearly, if one is at risk for skin cancer, it's important to make sun safety a priority. Doing so, however, requires some thought—and it often means confronting the fact of one's own risk—which is not always a pleasant task. It also takes time to apply sunscreen, wear protective clothing, and examine one's skin regularly for signs of skin cancer. Yet these are all important steps in protecting oneself from overexposure to the sun.

Recently, as I was preparing to cover a medical conference at the Moscone Convention Center in San Francisco, I discovered that I had neglected to practice good sun safety. I had donned a scoop-necked sleeveless sweater under my tailored pantsuit in preparation for the conference. I sauntered toward the convention center—enjoying the 15-minute walk from the parking garage. However, when I got home, I was distressed to find that the makeup with sunscreen I apply everyday had not been enough to protect me from the sun.

Above my scoop-necked shirt, my skin was decidedly pink. That 15-minute walk had been enough to overexpose my sensitive skin to the sun. The next day, as I prepared to go on a hike with a friend, I applied sunscreen around my neck above my T-shirt. "I guess you can never be too careful!" I thought ruefully as I grabbed my water bottle and my cotton hat in preparation for our walk.

Most experts agree that merely applying sunscreen is not enough to protect you from skin cancer. Instead, what's needed is a four-pronged approach[11]:

- Limiting your time in the sun, especially during the hours of intense sunlight from 10 AM. to 4 PM.

- Wearing sun-protective clothing and sunglasses
- Using sunscreen with an SPF of at least 15 that protects from both UVA light and UVB light—two types of ultraviolet light that come from the sun—and applying it properly
- Avoiding tanning beds and sunlamps

What Are UVA and UVB Light and What's the Difference?

The sun produces sunlight, which we can see, as well as UV light. UV light rays are energy waves that are shorter in length than visible light rays. Because of this, the human eye cannot see UV light. UV rays are actually a type of radiation, and both UVA and UVB can pass through the earth's atmosphere and affect our skin. They both can cause skin damage and play a part in causing skin cancer. UVA penetrates into the deepest skin layers and causes damage to connective tissue there. UVA is linked mainly to some damage to cells' DNA that results in aging of the skin and wrinkles, but it is also thought to play a role in causing skin cancer. UVB rays penetrate less deeply into the skin than do UVA rays, but they cause direct damage to DNA and are responsible for sunburns. They're also thought to cause most skin cancers.[6,12,13]

When it comes to sun exposure, it's important to be careful. Sunlight is responsible for more than 90% of all nonmelanoma skin cancers and 65% of melanomas, according to the Skin Cancer Foundation.[1] You may be surprised to find that the U.S. Department of Health and Human Services actually classifies UV radiation as a carcinogen (a cancer-causing agent). UV light exposure also increases the likelihood of cataracts and suppresses the body's immune system.

It's thought that UV light causes changes in the DNA of several genes that regulate growth and survival of skin cells. Research suggests that some of these changes are caused by UVA and others by UVB and that damage to different genes seems to be more common in the three main forms of skin cancer (SCC, BCC, and melanoma). For example, damage to the *p53* gene, which normally suppresses cancer growth, seems to have an important role in SCC. "When there's a mutation in the *p53* gene, injured cells in the skin that normally would die off keep dividing instead. These abnormal cells then can lead to cancer," says David Leffell, MD,

Rules for Sun Protection

Many people think that they need to protect themselves from the sun only when they spend a day at the pool or beach. But sun exposure actually adds up day after day, so it's important to protect yourself from UV radiation whenever you expect to spend time outdoors. The American Cancer Society's catch phrase—Slip! Slop! Slap and Wrap!—can help you to remember the four most important approaches to sun protection. The slogan stands for "Slip on a shirt. Slop on sunscreen. Slap on a hat, and wrap on sunglasses to protect your eyes and the skin around them from the sun." Here are some tips for following these practical rules for sun protection:

- *Cover up with clothing.* Long-sleeved shirts and long pants or skirts are the most protective, and dark colors are better than light colors. Tightly woven dry fabric provides more sun protection than fabrics that are wet or loosely woven. One good rule of thumb: If you can see light through a fabric, UV rays can get through, too. Some companies now make sun-protective clothing—usually tightly woven or with special coatings that help absorb UV rays. The higher the UV protection factor (UPF) listed on the label, the more it protects you from the sun's rays.

- *Apply sunscreen.* Remember, however, that it doesn't provide total protection from the sun. Use sunscreen with an SPF of at least 15 or higher. To get benefit from sunscreens, apply them properly! It's important to smooth the sunscreen on dry skin 20 to 30 minutes before going outside to give it time to absorb into the skin. Use at least a palm full or 1 ounce of sunscreen to cover your arms, legs, neck, and face if you are an average-size adult. Reapply it every 2 hours after you get outdoors. Those labeled "waterproof" actually provide protection for only 80 minutes when swimming or sweating, and those labeled "water resistant" protect for only 40 minutes. After swimming, sweating, or toweling yourself dry, therefore, you'll need to reapply your sunscreen.

- *Cover your head with a hat.* Hats that have at least a 2- to 3-inch brim around—not just at the front—give the most protection from the sun. They'll protect areas such as your forehead, nose, scalp, neck, and ears. Another good choice is a shade cap (with about 7 inches of fabric that drapes down the back and sides). A baseball cap protects only the front and top of the head but not the back of the neck or ears, where skin cancers are likely to develop. Straw hats are not wise choices either, unless they're tightly woven.

- *Wear sunglasses that protect the skin around your eyes from UV rays.* Long hours in the sun not only lead to skin cancer but also can result in an increased risk of cataracts and some other eye disease. UV-blocking sunglasses block 99% to 100% of UVA and UVB radiation. Some labels on sunglasses will say "UV absorption up to 400 nm," which is the same as 100% UV absorption. Those with labels that say "Meets ANSI UV requirements" block 99% of the sun's rays, whereas those labeled "cosmetic" block only 70% of the sun's rays. Dark glasses are not necessarily better because the UV protection comes from a chemical applied to the glasses, not from the darkness or color. Finally, large-framed or wrap-around sunglasses are the most likely to protect your eyes from sun coming in at different angles.

—From "How Do I Protect Myself from UV?" American Cancer Society[20]

professor of dermatologic surgery at Yale University. He notes that studies have shown that sunscreen can help to prevent the mutation in the *p53* gene that can lead to skin cancer.

In my early 30s, I worked as a newspaper reporter at the *Houston Post* in Texas and had a chance to interview famed cancer researcher Margaret Kripke, PhD, of the University of Texas MD Anderson Cancer Center, whose work concerned the interrelationship of UV light and the immune system as a cause for skin cancer. As our hour-long interview came to a close, I asked Dr. Kripke a quick question: "What is the best hope for curing skin cancer?" Her answer was both considered and simple. "It's not to get it at all," she said. "You can't overemphasize the need for prevention. In my lab, the animals don't get skin cancer if I turn off the UV lights," she said.

The Sun and Vitamin D

Recently, news reports have highlighted the benefits of getting sun—or, at least, the benefits of getting enough sun exposure to boost your store of vitamin D. UV light, as well as being a cause of skin cancer, increases the skin's production of vitamin D. Recent studies have suggested that vitamin D can reduce the risk of colon, breast, prostate, and ovarian cancers. Recent headlines tell the story: "Vitamin D Benefits from Sun Exposure Outshine Cancer Risk" and "Cancer Meta-Analyses Shine on Vitamin D." So the question becomes: Should you increase your sun exposure to get vitamin D? Most dermatologists and oncologists say no, whereas some other researchers disagree.

In a study published in the prestigious *Proceedings of the National Academy of Sciences*[14] in 2008, researchers concluded that the benefits of increased sun exposure outweighed its risks. As well as protecting against several cancers, vitamin D seems to help reduce the risk of multiple sclerosis, bone diseases such as osteoporosis, and cardiovascular events, the researchers said. "These issues have health consequences far beyond those of cancer because a number of diseases are associated with inadequate vitamin D levels or low sun exposure: neurological, cardiovascular, metabolic, immune, and bone diseases," they noted. Some experts are also concerned that some people—particularly the elderly—are deficient in vitamin D, a problem that can lead to conditions such as osteopenia and osteoporosis, in which bones become more fragile and fractures can occur easily. Some of this research is beyond argument—there are many people who are deficient in vitamin D, according to experts. And we do know that getting sufficient vitamin D protects against bone conditions such as osteoporosis.

What *is* in question is how to get your vitamin D and how much benefit vitamin D confers when it comes to reducing cancer risk. Many dermatology experts are concerned that encouraging people to get more vitamin D from the sun will only worsen the epidemic of skin cancer. Also, not all studies agree that vitamin D is protective against cancers of the breast, colon, prostate, and ovaries. This research is in its preliminary stages, so it's too soon to be making health recommendations based on these particular findings. "The research on vitamin D is not accepted as dogma," Leffell says. "Most active people get enough UV radiation from the sun, and there's no need to increase it. It's also possible to get substantial vitamin D from supplementation."

"The problem is that once you tell people 'Oh, you can go out in the sun,' it becomes quite easy to overdo it," agrees Dr. Cockerell. "Everyone needs a little sunlight—but most people get enough without trying. In today's world, it's easy to get enough vitamin D from diet or supplements."

Safer ways to get enough vitamin D include your diet and supplements, as Leffell and Cockerell note. Dietary sources of vitamin D don't increase your risk for skin cancer or prematurely age your skin. And they're available year-round. Good dietary sources of vitamin D include fortified milk, fortified cereal, salmon, mackerel, and cod liver oil. Vitamin D supplements are well tolerated, safe, and effective.[15,16] The US Recommended Daily Allowance (RDA) for vitamin D is 400 International Units (IU). Although some experts say that this number should be raised, we do know that it is not safe to take more than 2000 IU per day. Supplements are a good way to get enough vitamin D, especially if you're worried that you're not getting sufficient amounts in your diet.

Human beings also need calcium to benefit from vitamin D, and sun exposure doesn't provide calcium. However, fortified milk, other fortified dairy products, and salmon are all rich in vitamin D and calcium. Many dietary supplements contain both—and getting enough calcium and vitamin D is crucial to preventing osteoporosis, the disease that results when the bones become more fragile and brittle as we age.

Remember that there is no easy rule or "one size fits all" prescription for the minimum amount of sun exposure that is needed to meet vitamin D requirements, according to the American Cancer Society. This is so because the amount of vitamin D our bodies make when exposed to sunlight will vary depending on age, skin color, time of day, how cloudy it is, the length of exposure and how much skin is exposed, and even geographic location. This is why it's more reliable—and safer—to get your vitamin D from diet or supplements.[16]

How Effective Is Sunscreen?

Many consumers might be surprised to learn that, for years, a debate has centered on the usefulness of sunscreens in preventing cancer. Some people have even suggested that sunscreens increase the risk for skin cancer. In truth, there are several possible explanations for reports claiming a link between sunscreens and skin cancer: Some people use sunscreens to prolong their time in the sun rather than to reduce their UV exposure, many use an inadequate amount of sunscreen to protect themselves from UV radiation, and use of sunscreen tends to be greatest in people with fair skin who are most susceptible to skin cancer.[17,18] Some of the strongest evidence that sunscreen use is safe and effective in preventing skin cancer comes from a randomized, controlled trial of 1621 adults living in Nambour, a subtropical Australian township. When compared with a group of adults who used sunscreen at their discretion, if at all, those who used broad-spectrum SPF-15 sunscreen daily had a 40% reduction in

SCC after 4.5 years. Eight years after the study was over, the risk for SCC continued to be 40% lower in the sunscreen group, and the rate of BCC also was 25% lower in the sunscreen group—although this number was not statistically significant. Why did the rate of cancers continue to be lower in the sunscreen group even though the trial had come to a halt? The sunscreen users may have learned the benefits of using sunscreen while enrolled in the trial, and their frequent use of sunscreen may have persisted to a greater extent than in the control group.[18,19]

However, some other scientists have suggested that blanket advice to the public to wear sunscreens at any time outdoors isn't warranted. The reason is that the relationship among sun exposure, sunscreen use, and the development of skin cancer is complex, and studies that have examined this relationship have not all found benefits for sunscreen use, particularly when it comes to melanoma. These studies are also limited by people's recall of their sun-exposure habits, including when and how much they've been sunburned, and difficulties in measuring and assessing the amount and frequency with which they use sunscreen.[17,18]

Most experts do agree, though, that by adopting a three-part strategy, you can reduce your UV exposure and your risk for skin cancer: limiting time in the sun, wearing protective clothing, and using sunscreens. Using these three tactics together provides the best opportunity to reduce your risk of skin cancer.

When used correctly, sunscreen with an SPF of 15—the minimum recommended by experts such as those at the American Academy of Dermatology and the American Cancer Society—deflects or absorbs 93% of the sun's UVB rays. However, most people don't use enough sunscreen to receive the level of protection that is indicated on the package. And most people fail to apply sunscreen at least 15 to 30 minutes before going outdoors, which allows the active ingredients to be completely absorbed into the skin, and they neglect to reapply sunscreen every 2 hours or after swimming.

The SPF number on most sunscreens reflects the product's ability to protect against UVB light—one of the types of light that comes from the sun. Within the last 20 years, it's also been recognized that another type of light that comes from the sun—UVA—acts as a carcinogen and also ages the skin. Newer sunscreens include UVA-blocking agents, such as avobenzone, ecamsule, zinc oxide, and titanium dioxide. For protection from both UVA and UVB rays, look for a sunscreen that is labeled "broad spectrum." Also check your sunscreen for the expiration date. Most are not effective after 2 to 3 years.[11]

The US Food and Drug Administration (FDA) has proposed a new regulation that would change the labeling on sunscreens to include protection against UVA. A four-star rating system would inform consumers about how well sunscreen products protect them against UVA light. "It's a good idea to look for products that protect against UVA—and to use a sunscreen with an SPF that is as high as possible. The idea is to maximize your protection from overexposure to UV rays," says Dr. Cockerell.

What Does SPF Mean?

The sun protection factor (SPF) rating on sunscreen is a measure of how much protection is provided against UVB rays. When you use an SPF-15 sunscreen and apply it correctly, you get the equivalent of 1 minute of unprotected UVB rays for every 15 minutes you spend in the sun. So, after 1 hour of wearing SPF-15 sunscreen, you'll have the same UVB exposure as someone who spent 4 minutes without protection from the sun. While sunscreens are available with SPFs as high as 100, it's important to remember that the higher the SPF number, the smaller is the difference between sunscreens. For instance, SPF-15 sunscreens filter out 93% of UVB rays, SPF-30 sunscreens filter out 97%, SPF-50 sunscreens filter out about 98%, and SPF-100 sunscreens filter out about 99%, according to the American Cancer Society. [20]

—From "How Do I Protect Myself from UV?" American Cancer Society

---

Tanning Beds and Skin Cancer

In addition to poor sun-protection habits in the outdoors, another trend that has scientists worried is the increasing use of tanning beds in our society. "One principal factor driving tanning behavior is the cultural belief that equates tanned skin with beauty and affluence. Tanning is no longer the mark of the common man, toiling outdoors for his living. Tanned skin is now viewed as a luxury: a sign that one can afford time away from the office," wrote Robert J. MacNeal and James G. H. Dinulos in a 2007 article in *Current Opinion in Pediatrics*.

Using indoor tanning as a way to achieve this view of beauty has become increasingly popular over the last 30 years. While the tanning industry has tried to downplay the risk, scientific evidence indicates that people who use tanning beds are at increased risk for skin cancer. For instance, using a tanning device doubles the risk of SCC and increases the risk for BCC by 50%, according to a 2002 study in the *Journal of the National Cancer Institute*. The younger you start using tanning beds, the higher is your risk for these cancers.[21] An important study published in 2007—a summary of 19 reports that evaluated the link between tanning beds and melanoma—found an increased risk for this cancer among those who tanned indoors. And those who used indoor tanning devices before age 35 had a 75% increased risk of melanoma.[22,23]

In 2009, the International Agency for Research on Cancer (part of the World Health Organization) elevated tanning beds to its highest cancer risk category—"carcinogenic to humans" (Group 1). Tanning beds previously had been classified as "probably carcinogenic to humans."[24]

Scientists and cancer advocates are especially concerned about the use of tanning beds among adolescents and teenagers. In the United States, most adolescents are aware of the harmful effects of UV radiation but continue to expose themselves to artificial and natural UV radiation without adequate protection, according to the American Academy of Dermatology. Yet sun exposure in the teenage years puts one at risk for cancer years later in adulthood.

Why would teenagers engage in such risky behavior? A study published in *Cancer Causes Control* in 2006 examined the use of tanning beds among teenagers and associated this use with other high-risk adolescent behaviors, such as drug use, binge drinking, and unhealthy weight loss.[25] Termed the "Growing Up Today Study," this study evaluated more than 6000 adolescent girls and their health behaviors. Other studies also have suggested an association between indoor tanning and risky behaviors that include alcohol, tobacco, and drug use.[4]

There is some thought that indoor tanning also can be addictive for some people. A high percentage of adolescents who tan have a difficult time quitting, according to a 2006 study in the *Journal of the American Academy of Dermatology*. These adolescents usually began tanning at early ages. Small studies also have reported that exposing oneself to tanning and tanning beds may be pleasurable—making it more difficult to quit. Tanning may increase the release of endorphins, the body's "feel good" chemicals, some researchers have speculated. In recent studies, when individuals were blindfolded and exposed to tanning beds with and without UV radiation filters, for instance, most preferred and chose unfiltered UV radiation.[4,26,27]

Many states have passed legislation that limits a minor's access to indoor tanning facilities. Some states prohibit the use of tanning facilities by children younger than age 15, whereas other states require older adolescents to have parental permission for indoor tanning. Yet, despite these regulations, studies show that many tanning facilities fail to bar underage children and those with photosensitive skin.[4]

Sunless tanners are a safer alternative to indoor tanning. Sunless tanners are cosmetic products that darken or stain the skin; their effects last for several days. However, they can cause rashes in some people and should not be used around the eyes. Sunless tanners don't cause cancer. Dihydroxyacetone is the ingredient in sunless tanners that darkens the skin. Previously, sunless tanners often produced an artificial and streaky appearance. Newer formulations provide natural-appearing colors and have gained wider acceptance. One important note of caution: Remember that using a sunless tanner will not protect you from sunburn or skin damage once you go out in the sun.[4,28]

Recognizing Skin Cancer Early

Many researchers believe that the best way to stop skin cancer in its track is to recognize it early. When skin cancer is localized, it has a high cure rate. However, finding skin cancer early means being aware of your moles and other skin markings and regularly doing a skin self-exam if you're at increased risk of skin cancer. If you've had skin cancer or think you may be at risk for the disease, it's important to do a skin self-exam at least once a month and to have a dermatologist check your skin every year.

Here's how to do a skin self-exam:

- Stand in a room with good light and a full-length mirror, and make sure that there's a handheld mirror nearby.

- With your clothes off, inspect your body for unusual moles or skin growths or discolorations in the full-length and handheld mirrors. The handheld mirror can help you to check your thighs, genital area, back, and scalp. It sometimes helps to do this both standing and sitting on a small stool or chair—just to make sure that you clearly see all parts of your body.

- Later, have a friend or your hairdresser scan your scalp for moles. This person can use a comb or blow dryer to move your hair out of the way.[8,28]

Signs of Melanoma

Melanoma *can* be caught early when it is most curable. The most important way to find melanoma early is to do regular skin exams and know
the patterns of moles, freckles, and blemishes on your skin. *One of the*
most important signs to watch for is a spot or mole that is new or one
that changes in size, feel, color, or shape.

It may appear as a new mole, look black or different from other moles
or spots on your skin, or may be "ugly looking." The mole may have fine
scales or may itch. The texture may change so that the mole becomes
hard and lumpy, or it may ooze or bleed. Moles that continue to change
over a month or more are of most concern. Any change in your skin
should be evaluated by a physician.

Most normal moles are evenly colored and are tan, brown, or black.
They may be raised, flat, oval, or round. They're generally less than the
width of a pencil eraser. Besides noting changes in spots or moles on
your skin, the ABCD rule can help you to recognize an abnormal mole or
melanoma. Moles with any of these characteristics should be evaluated
by your physician.[5,7,29]

- *Asymmetry*—the shape of half of a mole does not match the
  other half
- *Border*—the edges of the mole are irregular, ragged, notched,
  or blurred, and the pigment may spread into surrounding skin.
- *Color*—the color of the mole is uneven and can range from
  black to tan to brown. There may be areas of gray, white, red,
  pink, or blue.
- *Diameter*—the mole changes in size, usually increasing, and is
  usually larger than 6 mm, the size of a pencil eraser.

Signs of Nonmelanoma Skin Cancer

The most important signs of BCC or SCC are new growths, a bump or
spot that changes or gets larger over several months or years, or a sore
that hasn't healed within a period of 3 months. Other signs of BCC and
SCC include[5,7]

BCC:
- Firm, flat, pale areas on the skin
- Small, raised, red or pink areas that are waxy, shiny, and/or
  bleed after minor injuries

- Spots with blue, black, or brown areas, a depressed center, or visible blood vessels
- Large spots that ooze or have crusts

SCC:

- Lumps that appear to be growing
- Bumps or lumps with a rough surface
- Flat red patches that grow slowly on the skin

What Are Actinic Keratoses?

Actinic keratoses are also referred to as *solar keratoses* and are found on chronically sun-exposed skin, most commonly on fair-skinned people. They are commonly found on the face and the backs of the hands. Actinic keratosis lesions are scaly flat growths that look like rough brown or red patches, and their size ranges from being as small as a pinhead to more than the size of a quarter. Another sign of actinic keratosis is peeling or cracking of the lips that doesn't heal. Without treatment, these growths can become SCC. You frequently can identify actinic keratoses by the way they look and feel—as rough as sandpaper.[8,30]

Resources

American Cancer Society Fact Sheet on nonmelanoma cancer:
www.cancer.org/docroot/CRI/CRI_2x.asp?sitearea=&dt=51

American Cancer Society Fact Sheet on melanoma skin cancer:
www.cancer.org/docroot/CRI/CRI_2x.asp?sitearea=&dt=39

National Cancer Institute information on nonmelanoma skin cancer:
www.cancer.gov/cancertopics/types/skin

National Cancer Institute information on melanoma:
www.cancer.gov/cancertopics/types/melanoma

The American Academy of Dermatology:
www.aad.org

The Melanoma Research Foundation:
www.melanoma.org

The Foundation for Melanoma Research:
  www.foundationformelanomaresearch.org
The Skin Cancer Foundation:
  www.skincancer.org

References

1. The Skin Cancer Foundation. *Skin Cancer Facts*. Available at www.skincancer.org/Skin-Cancer-Facts. Accessed July 14, 2009.

2. NCI SEER Cancer Statistics. Available at http://seer.cancer.gov/statfacts/html/melan.html and www.cancer.gov/cancertopics/types/skin. Accessed July 14, 2009.

3. American Cancer Society. *Cancer Facts and Figures 2009*. Atlanta: American Cancer Society; 2009.

4. MacNeal RJ, Dinulos JGH. Update on sun protection and tanning in children. *Curr Opin Pediatr*. 2007;19:425–429.

5. American Cancer Society. *Detailed Guide: Skin Cancer–Melanoma*. Available at www.cancer.org/docroot/CRI/CRI_2_3x.asp?dt=39. Accessed July 14, 2009.

6. American Cancer Society. *Detailed Guide: Skin Cancer–Basal and Squamous Cell*. Available at www.cancer.org/docroot/CRI/CRI_2_3x.asp?dt=51. Accessed July 14, 2009.

7. National Cancer Institute. *What You Need to Know About Melanoma*. Available at www.cancer.gov/cancertopics/wyntk/melanoma. Accessed July 14, 2009.

8. National Cancer Institute. *What You Need to Know About Skin Cancer*. Available at www.cancer.gov/cancertopics/wyntk/skin. Accessed July 14, 2009.

9. Leiter U, Garbe C. Epidemiology of melanoma and nonmelanoma skin cancer—the role of sunlight. *Adv Exp Med Biol*. 2008;624:89–103.

10. Kricker A, Armstrong BK, English DR, et al. Does intermittent sun exposure cause basal cell carcinoma? A case-control study in Western Australia. *Int J Cancer*. 1995;60:489–494.

11. American Cancer Society. *Skin Cancer Prevention and Early Detection*. Available at www.cancer.org/docroot/PED/content/ped_7_1_Skin_Cancer_Detection_What_You_Can_Do.asp. Accessed July 14, 2009.

12. Centers for Disease Control and Prevention. *Healthy Youth! Skin Cancer. School Health Guidelines. Questions & Answers on Skin Cancer Prevention*. Available at www.cdc.gov/healthyyouth/skincancer/guidelines/questions.htm. Accessed July 14, 2009.

13. The Skin Cancer Foundation. *UV Information*. Available at www.skincancer.org/shining-light-on-ultraviolet-radiation.html. Accessed July 14, 2009.

14. Moan J, Porojinicu AC, Dahlback A, et al. Addressing the health benefits and risks, involving vitamin or skin cancer, of increased sun exposure. *Proc Natl Acad Sci USA*. 2008;105:668–673.

15. The American Cancer Society. *Vitamin D*. Available at www.cancer.org/doc-root/ETO/content/ETO_5_3X_Vitamin_D.asp?sitearea=ETO. Accessed July 14, 2009.

16. American Academy of Dermatology. *Vitamin D Fact Sheet*. Available at www.aad.org/media/background/factsheets/fact_vitamind.htm. Accessed July 14, 2009.

17. Green AC, Williams GM. Point: Sunscreen use is a safe and effective approach to skin cancer prevention. *Cancer Epidemiol Biomarkers Prev*. 2007;16:1921–1922.

18. Berwick M. Counterpoint: Sunscreen use is a safe and effective approach to cancer prevention. *Cancer Epidemiol Biomarkers Prev*. 2007;16:1923–1924.

19. Van der Pols JC, Williams GM, Pandeya N, et al. Prolonged prevention of squamous cell carcinoma of the skin by sunscreen use. *Cancer Epidemiol Biomarkers Prev*. 2006;15:2546–2548.

20. American Cancer Society. *How Do I Protect Myself from UV?* Available at www.cancer.org/docroot/PED/content/ped_7_1x_Protect_Your_Skin_From_UV.asp?sitearea=&level=. Accessed November 27, 2009.

21. Karaga MR, Stannard VA, Mott LA, et al. Use of tanning devices and risk of basal cell and squamous cell skin cancers. *J Natl Cancer Inst*. 2002;94:224–226.

22. Schulman JM, Fisher DE. Indoor ultraviolet tanning and skin cancer: health risks and opportunities. *Curr Opin Oncol*. 2009;21:144–149.

23. International Agency for Research on Cancer Working Group on Artificial Ultraviolet Light and Skin Cancer. The association of use of sunbeds with cutaneous malignant melanoma and other skin cancers: a systematic review. *Int J Cancer*. 2007;120:1116–1122.

24. American Cancer Society. "Tanning Beds Pose Serious Cancer Risk, Agency Says." ACS News Center. Snowden RV. Available at www.cancer.org/docroot/NWS/content/NWS_1_1x_Tanning_Beds_Pose_Definite_Cancer_Risk_Agency_Says.asp. Accessed July 30, 2009.

25. O'Riordan DL, Field AE, Geller AC, et al. Frequent tanning bed use, weight concerns, and other health risk behaviors in adolescent females (United States). *Cancer Causes Control*. 2006;17:679–686.

26. Zeller S, Lazovich D, Forster J, et al. Do adolescent indoor tanners exhibit dependency? *J Am Acad Dermatol*. 2006;54:589–596.

27. Feldman SR, Liguroi A, Kucenic M, et al. Ultraviolet exposure is a reinforcing stimulus in frequent indoor tanners. *J Am Acad Dermatol*. 2004;51:45–51.

28. American Cancer Society. *Skin Cancer Prevention and Early Detection*. Available at www.cancer.org/docroot/PED/content/ped_7_1_Skin_Cancer_Detection_What_You_Can_Do.asp. Accessed July 14, 2009.

29. Weinstock MA. Public health messages regarding skin cancer. *J Invest Dermatol.* 2004;123:xvii–xix.

30. The American Academy of Dermatology. *What Are Actinic Keratoses?* Available at www.aad.org/public/publications/pamphlets/sun_actinic.html. Accessed July 14, 2009.

5

A Powerful Anticancer Strategy: Physical Activity, Nutrition, and Avoiding Obesity

Many people would like to hear that there's a magic formula for reducing cancer risk. If you just eat a certain food or take a certain supplement, then you're safe—right? Well, no. Besides not smoking (which we'll cover in Chapter 6), what are the best lifestyle choices to make to reduce cancer risk? The answer may surprise you. It's a three-part strategy that packs a powerful punch against cancer and other diseases. The best way to reduce cancer risk through lifestyle choices, most experts agree, revolves around three important precautions

- Attain or maintain a healthy weight throughout life.
- Eat a nutritious diet, with an emphasis on plant sources, such as vegetables and fruits. Choose whole grains instead of processed (refined) grains, and limit consumption of processed or red meats and alcohol.
- Adopt a physically active lifestyle.

It sounds simple right? Well it may sound simple, but, as many people can attest, making these three choices can require not only willpower but also time and energy. So it's no wonder that most people would rather hear about that one supplement or magic food that promises to chase away cancer for good!

Yet the fact is that, in recent years, the evidence that weight, nutrition, and exercise are linked to reducing cancer risk has become overwhelming. And of these three, getting down to a desirable weight is probably the most important in terms of avoiding cancer.

"Besides not smoking, the number one rule for reducing cancer risk—whether you're a cancer survivor or not—should be to get down to a healthy weight," says Wendy Demark-Wahnefried, PhD, RD, professor of behavioral science at The University of Texas MD Anderson Cancer Center in Houston. "A lot of people ignore this fact. They ask me, 'Can I take soy or wheatgrass?' But the answer to reducing cancer risk is much less exotic. It means reducing your energy intake to get to a desirable weight, as well as eating a diet with lots of nutrients—plant foods, unrefined foods, and lots of fruits and vegetables with limited amounts of sugar and fat."

A surprising fact: Obesity, poor nutrition, and physical inactivity together cause about as many deaths from cancer as smoking—about a third of all deaths from cancer.[1] A report from the American Institute for Cancer Research (AICR) released in 2008 emphasized the link among unhealthy diet, overweight and obesity, a sedentary lifestyle, and cancer.[2] Its conclusions made headlines. *One coauthor of the AICR report, Walter Willett, MD, DrPH, an epidemiologist from the Harvard School of Public Health, told CBS News: Obesity is now "approaching smoking as a cancer risk" and may one day surpass smoking as the number one cancer risk.* According to the American Cancer Society, overweight and obesity contribute to 14% to 20% of all deaths from cancer.[3]

The authors of the AICR report said that the scientific evidence was "convincing" in linking overweight and obesity to

- Cancer of the esophagus
- Pancreatic cancer
- Cancers of the colon and rectum
- Cancers of the endometrium
- Cancers of the kidney
- Postmenopausal breast cancer

Excess weight even may be linked to some of the less common cancers, such as multiple myeloma, leukemia, non-Hodgkin lymphoma, thyroid cancer, and melanoma, according to a 2008 study in the *Lancet Oncology*.[4] What's problematic is that being overweight and obese is an epidemic today. Two-thirds of the people in the United States are overweight or obese.[5] And that fact has public health experts worried. As the number of overweight and obese people increases, it's likely that cancer rates, as well as the rates of a number of other health conditions, such as diabetes and heart disease, will increase. Some interesting facts about the link between weight and cancer risk include

- Overweight and obesity rates in children have tripled since the 1980s.[6] From 2003 to 2006, 12% of children aged 2 to 5 years,

17% of children age 6 to 11 years, and 18% of adolescents age 12 to 19 years were obese.[7] This increases their chance of becoming obese adults and their cancer risk as adults.

- The more weight you put on, the greater your cancer risk. Being obese, as compared with just being overweight, puts you at greater risk for diseases such as cancer.
- For adults, overweight and obesity are often calculated using height and weight to obtain a number called the *body mass index* (BMI). For an adult, overweight is defined as a BMI between 25 and 29.9. Obese is defined as a BMI over 30. You can calculate your BMI, using your height and weight, at the Web site of the National Heart Lung and Blood Institute (www.nhlbi.nih.gov/guidelines/obesity/bmi_tbl.htm). Although the BMI is a useful measure, it is not always considered the "gold standard" when it comes to calculating overweight. Some people with more muscular body builds—such as athletes—will have a higher BMI, but their risk for associated disease is less than those who have more fat and less muscle.
- Certain cancers, particularly those of the breast, colon, and prostate, are more likely to be aggressive in those who are overweight and obese.
- Extra weight on the abdomen is particularly dangerous in terms of cancer risk; it increases the chance for colon cancer, according to the American Institute for Cancer Research.[8]

What is overweight and obesity? For an average-height woman or man, Table 1 shows how many pounds it takes to be overweight or obese.[5]

Table 1   Overweight and Obesity Statistics for Average-Height Women and Men

	Women			Men	
Height	Overweight Pounds	Obese Pounds	Height	Overweight Pounds	Obese Pounds
5 ft, 2 in	136–163	164+	5 ft, 8 in	163–196	197+
5 ft, 3 in	141–168	169+	5 ft, 9 in	169–202	203+
5 ft, 4 in	145–173	174+	5 ft, 10 in	174–208	209+
5 ft, 5 in	150–179	180+	5 ft, 11 in	179–214	215+
5 ft, 6 in	155–185	186+	6 ft, 0 in	184–220	221+

The Story of Obesity: Why Is It So Bad for Us?

Obesity is thought to affect cancer risk in a number of ways. Yet the biological mechanism that explains why being overweight or obese is linked to cancer risk may be different for different cancers, according to the National Cancer Institute (NCI).

It's thought that obesity may cause alterations in or raise levels of sex hormones, such as estrogen, progesterone, and androgens, or contribute to changes in insulin-like growth factor 1 (IGF-1), a hormone that regulates cell growth and development. Obesity also may increase levels of insulin. These changes may account for the increased risk of cancers such as those of the breast, endometrium, and colon seen in people who are obese.

Proteins that help to make hormones less or more available to our body tissues, including sex hormone–binding globulin, also may be involved in increasing cancer risk in those who are obese. Obesity is also thought to affect the immune system, the body's protective defense against disease, according to the NCI and the American Cancer Society's guidelines on nutrition and physical activity, published in the journal *CA* in 2006.[1,8,9]

Why Is Obesity So Prevalent?

Although most people want to maintain a healthy lifestyle and stay at a healthy weight, that task may be difficult in today's society. We live in what some experts have termed an "obese-ogenic" environment, that is, a society that may promote obesity. There are some substantial barriers today to achieving healthy nutrition and an active lifestyle—all of which contribute to the obesity epidemic. For instance, portion sizes in restaurants have grown increasingly large in recent years. Consider those giant cookies available at coffee shops and grocery stores—they're packed with excess fat as well as a whopping amount of calories. An increasing number of households with multiple wage earners as well as long work hours means that there's also less time for preparation of healthy meals, and more families rely on unhealthy fast foods or processed foods to save time.[1]

More people spend increased time at sedentary work and less time at leisure, meaning that there's less time available and fewer opportunities for physical activity. Increased use of automobiles and the easy access to communications media such as television and computer games all promote a sedentary lifestyle. Neighborhoods where there's less access to sidewalks and parks also contribute to the obesity epidemic. This is particularly true in the inner cities, where it may feel unsafe to walk outdoors at night or for children to play outdoors. In today's hard economic times, physical education programs in schools have become a lower priority, so many children lose their access to group sports and physical activities during the daytime.[1]

Hopefully, community policies that promote good nutrition and physical activity, such as the establishment of outdoor farmers' markets and community gardens (where fresh fruits and vegetables are readily available) in inner cities, school lunch modifications, nutrition education, physical activity interventions, and increased funding for physical education in US schools, may help to encourage healthy lifestyles.

The Weight Loss Struggle

Many of us don't find it easy to stay at an ideal weight. I've struggled with my weight for years. When I turned 50, I realized I had to do something about my 30-pound weight gain over the past few years, when I was diagnosed with mild obstructive sleep apnea.

Obstructive sleep apnea is caused by a blockage of the airway during sleep, usually when the soft tissue in the rear of the throat collapses and the airway closes. It's more common in people who are overweight or obese. Sleep apnea affects 12 million Americans, and untreated, it can cause high blood pressure and cardiovascular disease, memory problems, weight gain, impotence, and headaches. And, of course, as a medical writer, I knew that my excess weight put me at increased risk of developing cancer, as well as heart disease and diabetes.

And, to tell the truth, the 30 pounds that I had put on over the last 2 years did not make me want to look in the mirror. I wanted to feel fit, as well as look good. And I wanted to do my best to avoid the cancer history of my mother and father, and losing weight was one way to accomplish that goal.

Luckily, I had a partner in weight loss—my husband. He had been diagnosed with severe sleep apnea and was as long overdue for a diet as I was. We decided on a program that combined personalized attention with easy-to-fix meals (because we were remodeling our kitchen) and settled on the Jenny Craig diet plan. I have to say that when the counselor at Jenny Craig took my "before" photo, I was shocked. Was that really me—that overweight woman in that photo? It was.

Going on a diet was an adjustment. The portion sizes of the Jenny Craig meals, albeit augmented with lots of fruits and vegetables, were *so small* compared with what I was used to eating. But I persisted in the diet—as well as exercising, hiking, dancing, and working out on a stationary bike. The weight loss has come slowly—a pound or two a week. Four months into the diet, I'm about halfway to my weight-loss goal. I'm more fit and have more energy than before embarking on my weight-loss plan, as well as feeling better about how I look. I also feel better about my risk for cancer—the more weight I lose, I know, the less risk I have. Although my family history of cancer is not something I can change, I can have an impact on my weight, diet, and exercise habits. And that can only increase my odds for avoiding the disease.

There are actually a number of strategies for losing weight, and what works for you is often an individual matter. For more information on incorporating healthy behavior changes, such as diet, nutrition, and exercise, into your lifestyle, see our "Conclusion: Putting It All Together."

What is the best way to lose weight? There are a lot of diet plans out there—and believe me, I've tried a lot of them. Some popular diet plans, such as Atkins and South Beach, restrict carbohydrates, whereas others, such as Weight Watchers, decrease portion sizes; others, such as the Dean Ornish diet, recommend vegetarian fare. The truth is, however, that all these diet plans work because they restrict calories, as well as recommend an increase in exercise. No matter which plan you choose, a diet plan works most effectively when you expend more energy (through exercise) than the calories you take in as food. Many experts agree that no matter what diet plan you choose, there are several simple steps that make weight loss easier. The important ingredients for weight loss include[1,8,10]

- *Replace high-calorie foods that have added fats and sugars with vegetables and fruits, whole grains, beans, and low-calorie beverages.* High-calorie foods with added fats and sugars include fried foods, cakes, cookies, candy, soft drinks, and ice cream. These foods are especially prevalent at fast-food restaurants, where meals are often high in calories and also may contain hidden fats. Fast-food meals are usually low in fruits, vegetables, beans, and whole grains, according to the American Cancer Society guidelines on nutrition and physical activity.[1]
- *Reduce your intake of foods with added saturated and trans fats and sugars, as well as alcohol.* They tend to provide a lot of calories without essential nutrients, according to the American Cancer Society.[1]
- *Limit your intake of energy-dense foods, that is, foods that have a lot of calories per ounce.* For example, steak has more calories per ounce and is more energy dense than

vegetable soup, according to the American Institute for Cancer Research.[8,10]

- *Balance your food and beverage intake with increasing physical activity.* This means reducing the calories you take in and increasing physical activity that burns calories. To lose weight, most people need to reduce their food intake by about 500 calories a day, according to the American Cancer Society guidelines on nutrition and physical activity. Also try to get up to 60 to 90 minutes of moderate to vigorous intensity physical activity every day.[1]

- *Limit portion sizes but cut back gradually.* If you try to lose weight but end up hungry, you're more likely to abandon your diet and overeat by snacking on high-calorie foods, according to the American Institute for Cancer Research.[8,10]

- *Monitor your food intake and level of activity.* This may mean keeping a food and activity diary and logging what you eat each day as well as how much physical activity you get, according to the American Cancer Society.[1] This tactic enables you to see where your problems are—in eating or exercise habits or both—and to see where you may need to make changes. (See "Conclusion: Putting It All Together" for more on making behavioral changes for good health.)

All well and good, but what if you find it difficult to follow any diet, even one with low energy density? Or you try every diet out there and still can't lose weight?

It's no secret that losing weight can be difficult—and maintaining that weight loss is even more difficult. In fact, losing weight and maintaining that lost weight is harder than just staying at a healthy weight. Some people may find losing weight almost impossible. They may have tried fad diets and supplements—weight-loss approaches that are ineffective and also unsafe. Genetics or a medical condition, such as thyroid disease, may complicate efforts at losing weight, in which case a consultation with a health professional may be needed to address underlying health conditions, as well as weight issues.

Yet, even if you can't lose that extra weight, there are ways to use nutrition and activity to lower your cancer risk. These include increasing the amount of plant foods in your diet and limiting red meat and processed meat, which are thought to contribute to cancer risk. A coach or trainer also may help in putting together a physical activity program that can reduce your risk of developing cancer—and may even lead to gradual weight loss by itself.

A Conversation With Thomas Sellers, Cancer Researcher

Thomas Sellers, PhD, MPH, executive vice president and associate director of the Cancer Prevention and Control Division of the Moffitt Cancer Center, is a researcher who is one of the leading experts on the link between obesity and exercise and cancer risk, particularly breast cancer risk. We posed a few questions to Dr. Sellers to get his viewpoints on these important subjects.

Q: *In terms of reducing cancer risk, does it matter at what age you lose weight?*
Dr. Sellers: It's never too late to lose weight, and the more one is able to attain an ideal weight for their height, the better. But it's not losing weight that's so difficult; it's maintaining that weight loss over time that's a challenge for many people.

Q: *How does exercise reduce cancer risk?*
Dr. Sellers: There may actually be a number of mechanisms by which exercise reduces cancer risk. Exercise decreases cancer risk because it leads to weight loss, but it also causes changes in the immune system, as well as changes in the levels of circulating hormones, such as estrogen. Of course, there may be other mechanisms that remain to be discovered.

Q: *To reduce cancer risk, what's the better bet: losing weight or exercise?*
Dr. Sellers: Exercising and dieting are both beneficial because they help you to lose weight or maintain ideal weight. Your metabolism changes when you exercise, and that helps you to lose weight, thus reducing cancer risk. In humans, exercise is also beneficial even when weight is not lost. But in animals the effect of calorie restriction seems to be independent of exercise. In fact, calorie restriction may be more powerful than exercise.

Q: *Can losing weight reduce breast cancer risk?*
Dr. Sellers: There are some published studies that indicate that losing weight can reduce breast cancer risk. In a paper we published in 2004, we investigated the association of weight change with breast cancer risk in the Iowa Women's Health Study (a study of 41,837 Iowa women aged 55 to 69 years begun in 1986 to determine whether diet, body fat distribution, and other risk factors were related to cancer incidence). We found that women who lost weight had a 70% decreased risk of postmenopausal breast cancer compared with those who gained weight over a period of 15 years. Women who reached a certain weight and then stopped gaining—or their weight leveled off—had a reduced risk of breast cancer

as well compared with women who followed the pattern most commonly observed here in America—where weight continues to go up with age.

Q: *Is obesity a risk factor for breast cancer at any age?*
Dr. Sellers: The influence of obesity on breast cancer may actually vary depending on whether you're talking about premenopausal or postmenopausal breast cancer. Overweight and obesity are not significant risk factors for premenopausal breast cancer but are for breast cancer after menopause (when most breast cancers occur).

Q: *Is there an increased risk for breast cancer associated with overweight, no matter when the weight is gained?*
Dr. Sellers: The current evidence suggests that what's important in cancer risk is the lifetime pattern and the rate of change in obesity. In other words, the greater the increase in weight, the greater is the risk for postmenopausal breast cancer. There are limited data that show that when the weight is gained actually makes a difference.

What About Specific Foods?

Are some foods extra healthy? Are there those that contribute to causing cancer? According to the AICR report, nonstarchy vegetables, fruits, and foods containing dietary fiber can provide protection against cancer. Vegetables and fruits may be especially important because they contain beneficial minerals, fiber, vitamins, and a variety of other substances that protect against a variety of cancers. Studies also have shown that individuals whose diets are low in fruits and vegetables and high in red and processed meats have an increased risk of the most common cancers, according to the American Cancer Society guidelines on nutrition and physical activity published in *CA*. Read on and discover the impact that foods have on cancer risk. But keep in mind that eating one particular kind of food is less likely to significantly protect against cancer than is eating a variety of healthy foods. Rather, it's the healthiness of your entire diet that's most important. According to the American Cancer Society Guidelines and the AICR report[1,2]:

- *Nonstarchy vegetables*, including green leafy vegetables such as spinach, vegetables in the cabbage family (such as broccoli and cabbage), peppers, tomatoes, carrots, and allium vegetables (such as garlic and onions), protect against cancers of the *mouth, pharynx, larynx, esophagus*, and *stomach*, according to the AICR report. Some scientific evidence also suggests that vegetables may help one to stay at a healthy weight, according to the American Cancer Society guidelines on nutrition and physical activity.[1] Those who eat more vegetables, as well as fruits, have less weight gain and a lower risk for obesity. But stay away from vegetables that are fried or those with calorie-dense sauces; they won't help you to avoid weight gain or obesity.[1] (For more on American Cancer Society guidelines on nutrition and physical activity, see the American Cancer Society Web site.) Fruits help to guard against cancers of the *mouth, pharynx,* and *larynx* and cancers of the *esophagus, lung,* and *stomach,* according to the AICR report. Like vegetables, they also help you to maintain or lose weight. High-calorie fruit juices, however, are not beneficial. They work against the goal of staying *at a healthy weight.*[1]

- *Foods high in fiber,* including whole-grain cereals, fruits, vegetables, and beans, may reduce the *risk of colon* cancer, according to the AICR report. *Whole grains* such as brown rice and whole-grain breads, pasta, and cereals also contain vitamins and minerals that have been linked to a lower risk of cancer in general, according to the AICR report and the American Cancer Society.

Are There Foods to Avoid in Terms of Cancer Prevention?

In a word, yes. If you want to reduce your risk of cancer, it's best to limit your intake of[1,2,8]

- Red meats, such as beef, lamb, and pork, and processed meats, such as hot dogs, ham, bologna, bacon, and sausage. Diets high in red meat and processed meats may be a cause of *colorectal cancer,* according to the AICR report. They also may increase risk for cancers of the rectum and prostate, according to the American Cancer Society.[1] It's thought that red meat contributes to cancer risk in a variety of ways. When you cook meat at high temperatures or on a grill, (for suggestions on healthy grilling, see box on page 73) carcinogens are produced. The iron content in red meat also may generate damaging free radicals in the colon. Substances that are used to process meats (including salt and nitrates) also may damage DNA, and the fat in meat may increase the concentration of bile acids in the stool that can promote cancer, according to the AICR and the American Cancer Society guidelines on nutrition and physical activity.

- Foods with high amounts of salt and foods processed with salt (or salt cured) have been implicated in *stomach cancer*, according to the AICR report.
- Alcohol. If you do drink alcohol, limit your intake to two drinks a day for men and one drink per day for women. Drinking alcohol, especially heavy drinking, can be a cause of cancers of the *mouth, pharynx, larynx, esophagus, liver, breast, colon*, and *rectum*, according to the AICR report and the American Cancer Society. Overall, total alcohol consumption, not the type of alcoholic beverage, is what matters when it comes to the link with cancer. Yet even a moderate intake of alcohol may confer some increased risk for breast cancer—especially in women who do not get enough folate. Regular consumption of even a few drinks a week is associated with an increased risk for breast cancer. At the same time, moderate alcohol intake also protects against heart disease because of its positive effects on high-density lipoprotein (HDL "good") cholesterol. In deciding whether or not to drink alcohol (in moderation), women should consider their possible risk for heart disease as well as breast cancer. Women at high risk for breast cancer might reasonably consider not drinking alcohol at all.[1]

Healthy Grilling Tips

To minimize your exposure to carcinogens while grilling meat outdoors, follow these tips from the American Cancer Society[11]:

- Choose lean cuts of meat, and trim the meat of any excess fat. Fat dripping onto hot coals causes smoke that contains potential carcinogens. Less fat means less smoke.

- Line the grill with foil, and poke small holes in it so the fat can still drip off, but the amount of smoke coming back onto the meat is less.

- Precook meats ahead of time in the microwave so that they don't have to sit on the grill as long.

- Avoid charring meat or eating parts that are especially burned and black.

Preparing Vegetables: The Facts About Cancer Risk

To reduce cancer risk, your body needs the nutrients available in healthy foods such as vegetables. But are raw vegetables better for us? And does cooking reduce the protective effect of many nutrients in vegetables? Raw vegetables actually have more healthy nutrients than cooked ones. Yet, although cooking reduces the total amount of nutrients in vegetables, it also increases the *bioavailability* of those nutrients, or their ability to be absorbed by the body, according to the AICR report. For instance, the phytochemicals called *carotenoids* (found in most vegetables, especially red or orange vegetables) can be absorbed more easily by the body when the vegetables are cooked or pureed or when oil is added. In a similar fashion, the phytochemical called *lycopene* found in tomatoes is absorbed more easily when the tomatoes are processed, so you get more lycopene from tomato paste than from tomatoes. Crushing tomatoes or cooking them or including them in foods with oil also seems to increase lycopene bioavailability.[2]

Nutrition, Supplements, and Cancer Risk

There are certain foods—including soy and tea—that have been widely publicized as reducing cancer risk. However, in truth, the evidence regarding the power of these foods to protect against cancer is mixed. In essence, different studies have come up with widely varying conclusions about the ability of soy and tea to protect against cancer. Also controversial is the subject of certain *ingredients* in foods that may protect against cancer risk, including the phytochemicals beta-carotene (found in red-orange vegetables and fruits) and lycopene (found in tomatoes and tomato-based foods).[8]

Let's examine these foods and ingredients one by one based on the American Cancer Society guidelines on nutrition and physical activity.[12]

Soy

Soy contains phytochemicals called *isoflavones* that may protect against cancers that are hormone-dependent, that is, cancers that seem to occur more often and more aggressively with the release and production of hormones such as estrogen and testosterone. These include breast and prostate cancer. Some studies have found a reduced risk of breast cancer in certain populations, such as in China, where people have high intakes of soy foods over many years. In December 2009, a study of 5042 breast cancer survivors in China published in the *Journal of the American Medical Association*[13] also found that those with the highest soy food intake had a decreased risk of recurrence. However, other studies have not found the same protective effect of soy foods—partly because soy intake in the United States is much lower than in countries such as China, and the types of soy foods consumed in China may provide more isoflavones.[14] Another consideration in interpreting the recent report is that it is likely that Chinese women have regularly consumed soy throughout their lifetime, whereas in the United States, consumption is much less common. We don't know whether starting to eat soy regularly after a cancer diagnosis would have the same effect as having a lifelong diet high in soy foods.

However, the idea of consuming high doses of soy additives or supplements to protect against cancer is controversial. Some researchers think that this choice has the potential to actually *increase* the risk of estrogen-dependent cancers, such as breast and endometrial cancer.

The reason? When ingested, soy releases weak estrogens that may be associated with some cancers. This caution is particularly true for breast cancer survivors, according to the American Cancer Society. The American Cancer Society advises breast cancer survivors *not to take soy-containing pills, powders, or supplements.* Consuming soy foods as part of a healthy plant-based diet is fine, though. When consumed in moderate or plentiful amounts as part of a healthy diet, soy foods are not harmful and may have a protective effect against breast cancer recurrence.[14]

Tea

Some researchers have found that tea does protect against cancer because of the antioxidants it contains. In animal studies, teas—especially green teas—have been shown to reduce cancer risk. However, studies in humans have had mixed results. Some have found that tea has a protective effect against cancers, whereas others have not.

Beta-Carotene

The antioxidant beta-carotene is found in many fruits and vegetables, and because fruits and vegetables are associated with a lower risk of cancer, it may seem plausible that taking high doses of beta-carotene might protect against the disease. Yet the results of three large clinical trials have found just the opposite. In two studies in which people took high doses of beta-carotene supplements, cigarette smokers were found to have an increased risk of lung cancer. A third study found that beta-carotene supplements did not have a protective effect, nor did they increase the risk for cancer. Some studies also have found that people who take beta-carotene supplements have an increased risk of all-cause mortality—that is, death from all causes overall, not just cancer.[15]

Lycopene

Lycopene is found primarily in tomatoes and tomato-based foods, as well as in pink grapefruit and watermelon to a lesser extent. Several studies have reported that consumption of tomato-based foods reduces the risk of some cancers. Yet researchers are not certain whether it is the lycopene that is responsible for the protective effect or some other nutrient in tomatoes, grapefruit, and watermelon. Currently, taking lycopene supplements is not advised.

Calcium

Several studies have found that foods that are high in calcium may help to protect against colorectal cancer. Calcium supplements do slightly reduce the chance for formation of colorectal adenomas, growths that can be precursors to colon cancer. However, there is also evidence that high calcium intakes are linked to increased risk for prostate cancer and to prostate cancers that are more aggressive. So it's wise to consume the recommended levels of calcium, largely through food sources. The recommended intake of calcium is 1000 mg a day for people aged 19 to 50 years and 1200 mg a day for people older than age 50. Calcium supplements often contain vitamin D as well, which has been found to be protective against breast and other cancers (see "Vitamin D" below). Foods that are good sources of calcium include low-fat dairy products and leafy green vegetables.

Folate

Folate is a B vitamin found in vegetables, such as leafy greens, peas, and beans; fruits such as oranges and strawberries; and enriched cereals and other grain products. Too little folate may increase the risk of cancers of the breast, colon, and rectum, particularly in people who drink alcohol. Current evidence suggests that to reduce cancer risk, folate is best obtained by eating vegetables, fruits, and enriched grain products. High-dose folate supplements do not seem to be protective against cancer, however.

Selenium

Selenium is a mineral that contributes to the ability of antioxidants to mount a defense against cancer. Some studies have shown that this mineral protects animals against cancer, and one experimental trial showed that selenium supplements may protect against cancers of the colon, lung, and prostate. However, a 7-year study of over 35,000 men at 427 centers in the United States—called the Selenium and Vitamin E Cancer Prevention Trial (SELECT)—published in 2009 showed that selenium did not protect against prostate cancer and also had no effect on lung, colorectal, or other cancers. The maximum dose of selenium should not be higher than 200 µg per day.[16,17]

Vitamin C

Many studies have linked consumption of vitamin C–rich foods with a reduced risk of cancer. Oranges, grapefruit, berries, and peppers are some of the foods that are high in vitamin C. Foods high in vitamin C may protect against cancer of the esophagus, according to the AICR report. However, when given as a supplement, vitamin C does not seem to protect against cancer. Until there's more proof that supplements can have a protective effect, it's best to get your vitamin C from the foods you eat rather than from high-dose supplements.

Vitamin D

A growing body of evidence suggests that vitamin D may help to protect against cancers of the colon and breast. However, keep in mind that this research has accumulated just over the past few years and, in terms of scientific evidence, is still in its early stages.

Vitamin D can be obtained through exposure to the sun (for about 15 minutes per day) and from oily fish, fortified foods such as milk and cereals, and supplements. There is growing concern among scientific experts that many Americans do not consume sufficient vitamin D to protect against cancer, as well as diseases such as osteoporosis, in which the bones become fragile and can fracture easily.

The current recommended levels of vitamin D are 200 to 600 International Units (IU) per day, but this may be inadequate, according to a growing number of scientists. Just what exactly is the optimal dose of vitamin D is still open to question, however. Some experts have proposed that levels as high as 1000 to 2000 IU are needed for an anticancer effect and to meet the needs of those who may be deficient in the vitamin— especially those with little sun exposure, the elderly, individuals with dark skin, and exclusively breast-fed babies (because breast milk does not contain vitamin D). Individuals with dark skin may be prone to vitamin D deficiency because their skin does not make as much vitamin D when exposed to the sun. Until more research is done on what may be the best intake of vitamin D, it's best to consider 2000 IU as the upper limit for vitamin D supplementation. To reduce the health risk associated with exposure to ultraviolet radiation, it's best to get vitamin D from a balanced diet, supplements, and by limiting sun exposure to small amounts.

Vitamin E

Vitamin E is a powerful antioxidant, but there are questions about whether it protects against cancer when taken as a supplement. One study has shown that smokers who took vitamin E had a lower risk of prostate cancer. Other data from a large study of male smokers showed that higher blood levels of alpha-tocopherol—the most active ingredient in vitamin E—were associated with a lowered risk of pancreatic cancer.[18] However, the evidence that vitamin E protects against cancer is sparse. The large SELECT trial, which studied the effects of vitamin E as well as selenium supplements on health outcomes, did not find that it protected against prostate cancer and had no effect on the risk of other cancers. Several studies and summary reports have shown no effect of vitamin E on increasing longevity or have revealed that taking these supplements actually increases premature death. [16,17]

Omega-3 Fatty Acids and Fish

Studies in animals have found that omega-3 fatty acids—found in fish and some seeds and nuts—may suppress cancer formation or hinder the progression of cancer. But there is limited evidence from scientific studies that consuming fish or omega-3 supplements has a benefit in terms of cancer risk. Certainly, eating fish rich in omega-3 fatty acids is associated with a reduced risk of cardiovascular disease, but keep in mind that some fish may have high levels of mercury, dioxins, polychlorinated biphenyls, and other environmental pollutants. Levels of these substances generally are highest in swordfish, tilefish, shark, and king mackerel. Women who are pregnant or planning to become pregnant and young children should not eat these fish.

The Bottom Line on Supplements

Most scientific experts recommend that it's best to get the nutrients that protect against cancer from a healthy diet. Although there is strong evidence that vegetables, fruits, and other plant-based foods may reduce cancer risk, there is not a lot of support for taking high-dose supplements to achieve the same goals. There is also evidence that high-dose supplements, particularly beta-carotene supplements, may increase lung cancer risk. Vitamin E also may increase the risk of heart failure and shorten life expectancy.

As noted earlier, the large 2009 SELECT trial also showed no benefit from vitamin E and selenium for preventing cancer.[17] A 2007 review of prior studies in the *Journal of the American Medical Association* also found that patients taking beta-carotene, vitamin A, and vitamin E alone or in combination with other supplements had a slightly shorter lifespan.[16]

Why do nutrients in foods seem to protect against cancer, whereas supplements with individual nutrients seem to have little effect on cancer risk or actually cause harm? The reason may be that the nutrients in food act together to produce the reduction in cancer risk. The individual substances available in pills may be only one of many substances responsible for the beneficial effects of whole foods, according to the American Cancer Society guide to nutrition and physical activity. Because there is some evidence of harm from high-dose supplements, and because the jury is still out on the benefits of such supplements, the AICR and the American Cancer Society recommend that nutritional needs should be met by diet alone. Some supplements, however, may be beneficial for some people, such as pregnant women and people with restricted dietary intakes. If you do take a supplement, the best choice is a balanced multivitamin that contains no more than 100% of the "Daily Value" of most nutrients.[1,2]

For more information on the role of specific foods and nutrients on cancer risk, see the American Cancer Society's publication *Common Questions About Diet and Cancer*, available on their Web site.

Being physically active is also vital for reducing cancer risk. In addition to helping to maintain a healthy weight or to lose weight, exercise has benefits apart from weight loss. It seems to have a beneficial effect on cancer risk, no matter what your weight is.

How does exercise decrease your cancer risk? There are a number of theories, and many scientists think that exercise reduces the production of hormones and proteins that stimulate growth in our cells. It also improves immune function. "We know that exercise collectively affects cancer risk, but there's also a gap in our understanding of exactly how it works to decrease risk," says Alpa Patel, PhD, strategic director of the Cancer Prevention Study 3 for the American Cancer Society.

Studies have revealed that regular moderate-intensity exercise or increased physical activity is associated with a reduced risk of several types of cancer, including breast, colon, prostate, and endometrial cancer. Scientific evidence indicates that at least 30 minutes of moderate or vigorous activity on 5 or more days per week can help to reduce cancer risk, although 45 to 60 minutes is ideal to reduce risk of some cancers, such as those of the colon and breast.[1] What's really exciting for cancer survivors is a series of new studies that show that exercise affects the risk of cancer recurrence. "There's a growing body of evidence that there's an increase in disease-free survival among cancer survivors who are physically active," Patel says. The benefits of exercise are especially

---

Why Does Exercise Decrease Your Cancer Risk?

Researchers think that exercise

- reduces the circulating levels of hormones such as estrogen that may feed tumor growth
- decreases body fat, which also lowers levels of circulating hormones
- improves insulin resistance, which has been linked to cancer risk
- speeds the passage of waste through the digestive system, lowering the risk of colon cancer
- improves immune function[8,19,20]

pronounced for those who are survivors of colon and breast cancer. Recent scientific findings indicate that women with a history of breast cancer who engage in 2 to 3 hours per week of brisk walking have a significantly lower risk of breast cancer recurrence and tend to live longer than women who are inactive. In the same way, men and women who are active after a diagnosis of colon cancer tend to have a better prognosis than sedentary survivors, according to a recent review of studies published in *Nature Reviews Cancer* in 2008.[19]

In addition to providing health benefits in terms of cancer prevention, exercise—especially if it's done with friends—is likely to have emotional and psychological benefits as well.

What kind of physical activity is protective? According to the experts, all types and levels of physical activity are protective against cancer. But the more physically active you are, the better.

The Payback of Exercise

Exercise, in addition to helping you to lose weight or maintain a desirable weight, also reduces the risk for developing

- Colon cancer
- Endometrial cancer
- Prostate cancer
- Postmenopausal breast cancer[1,2]

What Counts as Physical Activity?

Any type of activity is helpful in reducing cancer risk—but more vigorous activity is the most helpful. When you exercise, keep in mind that exercise intensity can be light, moderate, or vigorous (Table 2). Many types of physical activity can help to reduce cancer risk, not just aerobics at the gym or cycling on an exercise bike. Some examples of healthy and fun physical activities that can help to reduce cancer risk include bike rides, walking instead of driving, dancing, swimming, yoga, tennis, and golf (without a cart).[1,8]

For more information on food, nutrition, and physical activity, see the AICR's Web site at www.aicr.org or the American Cancer Society's *The Complete Guide—Nutrition and Physical Activity* at www.cancer.org.

Table 2   Levels and Types of Physical Activity

Exercise Intensity Level	Types of Physical Activity
Light	Slow walking, weeding the garden, light housework (such as dusting)
Moderate	Brisk walking (17-minute miles), leisurely cycling, dancing, slow swimming, using exercise equipment at a moderate pace, golf (without a cart), yoga, Tai'-chi, and Pilates
Vigorous	Running (10-minute miles), fast walking (12-minute miles), tennis, aerobic exercise classes, rapid cycling, climbing hills or stairs, basketball, squash, racquetball, dancing, gymnastics, rope skipping, and using exercise equipment at a vigorous pace

Source: Reprinted with permission from the American Institute for Cancer Research.

References

1. Kushi LH, Byerts T, Doyle C, et al. American Cancer Society Guidelines on Nutrition and Physical Activity for Cancer Prevention: Reducing the Risk of Cancer with Healthy Food Choices and Physical Activity. *CA Cancer J Clin.* 2006;56:254–281.

2. World Cancer Research Fund/American Institute for Cancer Research. *Food, Nutrition, Physical Activity and the Prevention of Cancer: A Global Perspective.* Washington: AICR, 2007. Available at www.dietandcancerreport.org/?p=ER. Accessed October 28, 2008.

3. American Cancer Society. *Cancer Facts and Figures 2009.* Available at www.cancer.org/docroot/STT/content/STT_1x_Cancer_Facts__Figures_2009.asp?from=fast. Accessed July 16, 2009.

4. Renehan AG, Tyson M, Egger M, et al. Body-mass index and incidence of cancer: a systematic review and meta-analysis of prospective observational studies. *Lancet Oncol.* 2008;371:569–578

5. Weight-Control Information Network, National Institute of Diabetes and Digestive and Kidney Diseases. *Statistics Related to Overweight and Obesity.* Available at http://win.niddk.nih.gov/statistics/. Accessed October 28, 2008.

6. Robert Wood Johnson Foundation. New Report Finds Obesity Epidemic Increases, July 1, 2009. Available at www.rwjf.org/childhoodobesity/product.jsp?id=45348. Accessed July 16, 2009.

7. Ogden CL, Carroll MD, Flegal KM. High body mass index for age among US children and adolescents 2003–2006. *JAMA.* 2008;299:2401–2405.

8. American Institute for Cancer Prevention. *Guidelines for Cancer Prevention.* Available at www.aicr.org/site/PageServer?pagename=pub_AICR_guidelines. Accessed July 16, 2009.

9. National Cancer Institute. *Obesity and Cancer: Questions and Answers.* Available at www.cancer.gov/cancertopics/factsheet/risk/obesity. Accessed July 16, 2009.

10. American Institute for Cancer Research. *Staying Lean for Cancer Prevention.* Available at www.aicr.org/site/PageServer?pagename=pub_guidelines_staying_lean_for_cancer_prevention. Accessed July 16, 2009.

11. American Cancer Society. *Healthy Grilling Tips.* Available at www.cancer.org/docroot/subsite/greatamericans/content/Healthy_Grilling_Tips.asp. Accessed July 25, 2009.

12. American Cancer Society. *The Complete Guide—Nutrition and Physical Activity.* Available at www.cancer.org/docroot/PED/content/PED_3_2X_Diet_and_Activity_Factors_That_Affect_Risks.asp?sitearea=PED. Accessed July 16, 2009.

13. Shu XO, Zheng Y, Cai H, et al. Soy food intake and breast cancer risk. *JAMA.* 2009;302:2437–2443.

14. Ballard-Barbash R, Neuhouser ML. Challenges in design and interpretation of observational research on health behaviors and cancer survival. *JAMA.* 2009;302:2483–2484.

15. American Cancer Society. *Common Questions about Diet and Cancer.* Available at: www.cancer.org/docroot/PED/content/PED_3_2X_Common_Questions_About_Diet_and_Cancer.asp. Accessed October 28, 2008.

16. Bjelakovic G, Nikolova D, Gludd LL, et al. Mortality in randomized trials of antioxidant supplements for primary and secondary prevention: systematic review and meta-analysis. *JAMA.* 2007;297:842–857.

17. Lippman SA, Klein EA, Goodman PJ. Effect of selenium and vitamin E on risk of prostate cancer and other cancers: the Selenium and Vitamin E Cancer Prevention Trial (SELECT). *JAMA.* 2009;301:39–51.

18. Stolzerg-Solomon R, Scheffler-Collins S, Weinstein S, et al. Vitamin E intake, α-tocopherol status, and pancreatic cancer in a cohort of male smokers. Abstract presented at the American Association for Cancer Research, San Diego, CA, April 12–16, 2008.

19. McTiernan A. Mechanisms linking physical activity with cancer. *Nat Rev Cancer.* 2008;8:205–211.

20. Medline Plus encyclopedia. Exercise and immunity. Available at www.nlm.nih.gov/medlineplus/ency/article/007165.htm. Accessed July 16, 2009.

6

Saving Your Life: Leaving Tobacco Behind

What did Peter Jennings, Desi Arnaz, and John Wayne have in common? They all died prematurely of lung cancer—deaths caused by tobacco use. The tragedy is that their premature deaths were preventable. Tobacco use is the most preventable cause of death in the United States.[1] In addition to being a cause of lung cancer, tobacco use increases the risk for a wide range of other cancers, including cancers of the mouth, pharynx, larynx, esophagus, stomach, pancreas, cervix, kidney, and bladder and acute myeloid leukemia, according to the National Cancer Institute. It also helps to cause a plethora of illnesses ranging from heart disease and stroke to emphysema and bronchitis.[2]

You don't have to be a smoker to suffer the ill effects of tobacco. Secondhand smoke has been implicated in thousands of lung cancer deaths in the United States each year, and some studies have connected it recently with sudden infant death syndrome in homes in which parents smoke.[3]

Yet, despite these facts, smoking remains a persistent habit in the United States. According to the National Institute on Drug Abuse, tobacco is one of the most widely abused substances in the United States. More than 20% of adults, or 44.5 million people, smoke cigarettes in the United States. Youth and adolescents are still picking up the tobacco habit, although there's been a decrease in smoking among the nation's adolescents and teens in recent years. One in five high school students smokes cigarettes, and 12% of middle school students use some form of tobacco.[3]

Most smokers, when surveyed, say that they want to quit, but only 4% to 7% are successful.[4] Why? Once started, the tobacco habit becomes psychologically and physically addictive. Even those diagnosed with cancer aren't always able to quit—despite the "wake-up call" of a cancer diagnosis. Of those diagnosed with lung cancer, for instance, a significant percentage—at least 13%—continue to smoke.[5] In the not too distant

> *Tobacco is the world's greatest weapon of mass destruction. It will kill more than 600 million people alive today—half of them children.*
> —John Seffrin, CEO, the American Cancer Society, May 2008

past, it was thought to be a waste of time to try to get those diagnosed with cancer to stop smoking. However, now we know that doing so not only may impact survival to some extent but also may improve quality of life.

My father was one of the unlucky ones. After developing a nagging cough, he quit smoking for good—after several unsuccessful attempts. He had been a heavy cigarette smoker for years. But, for my father, it was too late. He was diagnosed with lung cancer and had part of one lung

Some Facts About Smoking

- Lung cancer is the most common cause of cancer death among both men and women in the United States. About 90% of lung cancer cases are due to smoking.[2]

- Secondhand smoke exposure also causes 3000 lung cancer deaths each year in the United States.[6]

- Smoking kills 1/5 Americans—or an estimated 440,000 people in the United States each year through cancer, heart disease, emphysema, or other lung diseases.[3] More people die from smoking than from alcohol, cocaine, heroin, homicide, suicide, motor vehicle crashes, fire, and AIDS combined.[7] Wounds take longer to heal and the immune system may be less effective in smokers than in nonsmokers.[3]

- Men who smoke have a greater risk for sexual impotence or erectile dysfunction than nonsmokers. Short-term effects of smoking for both sexes include premature aging of the skin, a decrease in the ability to smell and taste, and stained teeth.[3]

surgically removed. Years later, he developed a second lung cancer, which metastasized to his bones.

Unfortunately, advertisements for tobacco don't portray the devastation that a tobacco habit can cause. In ads, TV series, and films that show smoking, smokers are often portrayed as fashionable and glamorous. But that wasn't the reality for either my father or my family. His death took away my second parent when I was 46 years old and caused me to descend into an emotional tailspin for several years. Although years before I had tolerated my friends' smoking habits, I now became a fervent believer in stop-smoking campaigns.

Even though my father's choice to stop smoking came too late for him, it may not be too late for those of you who smoke today. Just 2 weeks to 3 months after quitting, former smokers' circulation improves, and their lung function increases, according to the American Cancer Society. One year after quitting, the risk of coronary heart disease is cut in half. And 10 years after quitting, a former smoker's chances of lung cancer also decrease by 50%. The risk of developing other cancers, including mouth, throat, esophagus, bladder, cervix, and pancreatic cancer, is reduced substantially, too.[8]

What's so harmful about tobacco? More than 4000 chemicals are found in the smoke of tobacco products, some of them dangerous and known to contribute to cancer, including tar and carbon monoxide. These chemicals damage the inner walls of the arteries, leading to atherosclerosis. Atherosclerosis is a disease in which plaque builds up on the insides of your arteries (blood vessels that carry oxygen-rich blood to your heart and other parts of your body). Plaque is made up of fat, cholesterol, calcium, and other substances found in the blood and can harden and narrow your arteries—often leading to heart attack or stroke.

Nonsmokers exposed to tobacco smoke also inhale these dangerous chemicals.[9] In addition to inhaling the smoke exhaled by the smoker, they are also at risk of inhaling sidestream smoke—the more toxic smoke from the end of a burning pipe, cigar, or cigarette. Why is sidestream smoke more dangerous? When smokers inhale, the smoke leaves harmful deposits inside the body, but the lungs also act to partially cleanse the smoke before they exhale. Exhaled smoke actually contains fewer dangerous chemicals than sidestream smoke.[10]

So the more people smoke, the greater their risk for developing cancer, chronic bronchitis, heart disease, emphysema, and other illnesses. But even those who smoke only occasionally are at risk for these diseases. Low-tar cigarettes are also not safe. Studies show that when smokers switch to a low-tar cigarette, they are likely to inhale longer and more deeply to get the chemical they crave in tobacco—nicotine.[3]

Even those who don't inhale when smoking are at risk for developing cancer and tobacco-related illnesses. Instead of directly inhaling smoke from a cigarette, cigar, or pipe, they inhale it as secondhand smoke from the air around them. Cigar and pipe smokers, who often don't inhale at all, have an increased risk for tongue, mouth, lip, and a host of other cancers, including those of the lung, bladder, and pancreas. Whenever smoke touches living cells, it does harm, according to the American Cancer Society.[3]

The ingredient in tobacco that smokers crave is nicotine. When inhaled, nicotine in tobacco smoke rapidly reaches peak levels in the bloodstream and enters the brain. For cigar and pipe smokers and smokeless tobacco users, nicotine is absorbed through the mucous membranes of the mouth, throat, and nose and reaches peak levels in the blood and brain more slowly.[11,12]

Nicotine acts as a stimulant immediately after exposure because the chemical results in the discharge of epinephrine (or adrenaline). It also acts on brain pathways that regulate feelings of pleasure and increases the level of the "feel good" chemical dopamine. This is why smokers report a feeling of pleasure and calm when smoking. Yet nicotine dissipates rapidly within the body, as do the feelings of reward, which causes smokers to continue dosing to maintain their feelings of pleasure. Withdrawal symptoms include irritability, craving, problems with memory and attention, and increased appetite.[11-14] "Nicotine creates a demanding habit, a true physical need for smoking," says Frank Vitale, national director of the Pharmacy Partnership for Tobacco Cessation at the University of Pittsburgh School of Pharmacy.

The pleasurable feeling that comes from inhaling small amounts of nicotine and the physical withdrawal that occurs without this chemical are what make smoking such a difficult habit to quit. For some people, the sight, smell, and feel of a cigarette, pipe, or cigar—as well as the ritual of handling, lighting, and smoking—are all linked with the pleasurable aspects of smoking and can worsen cravings or withdrawals.[1]

However, the good news is that there are many therapies that can help with quitting smoking, including nicotine gum, patches, nasal spray, lozenges, and inhalers, as well as nonnicotine medications that can decrease cravings and other problems that crop up when quitting. Behavior therapies also can help smokers to address the environmental triggers for their smoking so that they can employ strategies to circumvent their urge to smoke.

When you do quit smoking, it is possible that you may gain weight. However, most smokers gain less than 10 pounds. And there are ways to reduce the chance that you'll gain weight. You can try a medication such

If You're a Smoker, Be Alert to These Symptoms

If you're a smoker, be sure to tell your healthcare providers so that they can help you to quit and provide preventive care for smoking-related health problems. The American Cancer Society recommends that periodic checkups for smokers should include mouth exams in order to prevent or find oral cancer early.

You should look for and alert your doctor if you notice any of the following symptoms:

- Any change in a cough, such as coughing up more mucus than usual
- A new cough
- Coughing up blood
- Hoarseness
- Trouble breathing
- Wheezing
- Headaches
- Chest pain
- Loss of appetite
- Weight loss
- Fatigue and feeling tired all the time
- Repeated respiratory infections

Any of these symptoms could be signs of a lung cancer or a number of other lung conditions. Keep in mind, however, that many lung cancers do not cause any noticeable symptoms until they are advanced and have spread to other parts of the body.

—From American Cancer Society, *Questions About Smoking, Tobacco, and Health*[3]

as bupropion (see discussion under "Preparing to Quit"), which tends to cut down on weight gain after you stop smoking, as well as helping to reduce symptoms of nicotine withdrawal. Other good ways to control your weight while quitting smoking are exercise and a healthy eating plan. Being physically active also may ease withdrawal symptoms during smoking cessation and help to reduce the chances of relapsing after quitting. And remember this important fact: If you're worried about weight gain, quitting smoking has many health benefits, and these benefits far outweigh any small weight gain.[15]

When a smoker quits, it is the nicotine withdrawal that leads to unpleasant symptoms. Nicotine-replacement therapy gives the smoker nicotine—in the form of gums, patches, sprays, inhalers, or lozenges—but not the other harmful chemicals in tobacco. Replacement therapy can help to relieve some of the symptoms of withdrawal so that a smoker can focus on the psychological aspects of quitting.[15] "Using nicotine-replacement therapies often keeps a smoker comfortable while they address the underlying reasons for their smoking habit," Vitale says.

Studies have shown that nicotine-replacement therapies—particularly the nicotine patch—even can be used safely by most smokers. The dose of nicotine you receive in nicotine-replacement products is small, and these products are also often used only for a short duration. Experts say that the benefits you get from successfully quitting smoking far outweigh any possible problems from nicotine-replacement products, even for those with cardiovascular disease—as long as they're monitored by a healthcare provider.[15]

However, nicotine-replacement therapy should not be the only method you use to quit smoking. Studies have shown that using nicotine-replacement products doubles the quit rate for smokers, but most of these studies also have included sustained behavioral support—counseling and support groups—for smokers.[16] Quitting smoking is not easy, and many people try many times before succeeding. Some people try hypnosis and other complementary and alternative medicine approaches to quitting smoking. "There are a lot of different products that can help smokers quit," Vitale says. "But using a nicotine-replacement therapy or a medication to stop smoking only addresses half the equation. It takes care of the physical addiction. To be successful, smokers have to address the feelings and events that make them want to smoke."

According to the Agency for Healthcare Research and Quality U.S. Preventive Services Task Force guidelines, combination therapy with medications (either nicotine-replacement therapy or the prescription medications discussed below) and behavioral counseling by addiction specialists or mental health professionals trained in addiction is more effective than either of these interventions alone.[17] Smoking-cessation methods that address the psychology and habit components of smoking are considered highly effective, particularly if the programs are sustained for four or more sessions, according to recent studies. These programs teach smokers ways to cope with smoking triggers and withdrawal symptoms, how to recover from slips and how to reach out for support from family and friends, and methods of preventing relapse.[18]

Smoking-Cessation Programs

A smoking-cessation program or class can be crucial to helping you quit. Not only do these programs give you advice about dealing with cravings, but they also provide emotional support and encouragement as well. They also can help you deal with problems that come up during quitting.

Studies have shown that the best programs include counseling, either one on one or in a group, led by someone trained in tobacco cessation. And there is a strong link between the intensity of the counseling and how successful people are at quitting. In other words, you have a greater chance of achieving your goal to quit with a more intense program.[19]

A more intense program usually means more sessions or longer sessions. The American Cancer Society recommends quit-smoking programs that are at least 20 to 30 minutes per session, contain at least four to seven sessions, and are held over at least 2 weeks.

In addition to stop-smoking classes run by the American Cancer Society or the local health department, many communities have Nicotine Anonymous groups that have regular meetings. There is no cost to attend. Nicotine Anonymous applies the principles of Alcoholics Anonymous to tobacco addiction.

According to the American Cancer Society, there are also some programs that are unethical and may not help you to quit. Steer clear of programs that

- Promise instant easy success with no effort on your part
- Use injections or pills with "secret" ingredients
- Charge a very high fee
- Are not willing to give you a reference from people who have used the program[15]

Tips to Help You Quit

To be successful at quitting smoking, you often have to change the behaviors that go along with smoking.

- When indulging in a behavior that was often linked with smoking, distract yourself by doing something different. If you had a cigarette after every meal, brush your teeth instead. Do a visualization—that is, bring to mind a pleasant visual image—in the morning on awaking instead of grabbing a cigarette, according to Vitale.
- If you miss the feeling of a cigarette in your hand, try holding something else—a pencil, coin, or marble, for example.[20]

- If you associate smoking with alcohol or coffee, try other drinks instead.[20]
- If you miss the feeling of a cigarette in your mouth, try cinnamon sticks, celery, or sugarless gum.[20]
- Stay away from situations you associate with smoking, and seek out public places where smoking is not allowed—libraries, museums, malls, and theaters.[20]
- Eat several small meals throughout the day to keep your blood sugar levels constant, which helps to prevent the urge to smoke.[20]
- If you feel that you're in danger of smoking, call a friend, family member, or a stop-smoking counselor.[20]

Preparing to Quit

There is no right way to quit smoking, but many smokers do prefer to quit cold turkey. If you do decide to go this route, it's best to pick a "Quit Day" and then stop smoking from that day on. You also also try smoking fewer cigarettes for 1 or 2 weeks before your "Quit Day." With this method, you can slowly reduce the amount of nicotine in your body. You can cut out cigarettes smoked with meals, or you could decide to smoke only at a certain time of the day. Although cutting down gradually often seems attractive to smokers, the truth is that it is often more difficult to quit this way.

Here are some suggestions from the American Cancer Society on how to set up a plan for not smoking[15]:

- Pick your "Quit Day," and mark it on the calendar.
- Tell your friends and family about your "Quit Day."
- Get rid of all the cigarettes, cigars, pipes, and ashtrays in your home, car, and place of work.
- Stock up on oral substitutes—including sugarless gum, carrot sticks, and hard candy.
- Decide on a plan. Will you use nicotine-replacement therapy or medications? Will you attend a stop-smoking class? If so, sign up now.
- Practice saying "No thank you. I don't smoke."
- Set up a support system. This support could be a group class, Nicotine Anonymous, or a friend or family member who has quit successfully and is willing to help. Ask family members and friends who smoke to not smoke around you and not leave cigarettes, pipes, or cigars out where you can see them.

- Think back on your previous attempts to quit. What worked and what didn't work for you? Identify the methods that were most effective for you.
- Another good technique for quitting smoking is to quit with a friend or partner.

Recent research by scientists funded by the National Institutes of Health shows that when people decide to quit, their spouses, family members, and friends are more likely to quit smoking, too. In the research, published in the *New England Journal of Medicine* in May 2008, close relationships had a definite influence on the decision to quit smoking, as well as the smoker's success in quitting. When a husband or wife quit smoking, it reduced the chance of their spouse smoking by 67%! And quitting smoking decreased the likelihood that friends would smoke by 36%. A similar effect on stop-smoking efforts was seen among coworkers at small firms, who often were influenced by fellow employees' decisions to quit.[21]

Another useful way to find support during the quitting process is to call an American Cancer Society *Quitline*. Many states run Quitlines through local health departments, and some corporations also have contracted with the American Cancer Society for their own Quitlines. Quitline is, simply put, a telephone-based stop-smoking counseling program. Since the American Cancer Society started providing Quitline services in 2000, it has served nearly 400,000 callers, according to J. Lee Westmaas, PhD, at the American Cancer Society.

The telephone counseling is provided in four to eight sessions. The Quitline counseling protocol is based on the principles of social cognitive theory, which says that people often learn best from role models whose behaviors they want to imitate. Quitline counselors are trained in providing motivational interviewing—that is, interviewing that encourages the smoker to quit—and cognitive behavioral therapy, a type of psychotherapy that focuses on changing behaviors and motivations associated with smoking, Dr. Westmaas says. The Quitline counselor will help you to select a "Quit Date" and then will follow up with two to three calls before your "Quit Date" and two to five calls afterward. By calling a Quitline, you can find individualized counseling and have the opportunity to ask any questions you have about quitting smoking. The American Cancer Society Quitline also provides self-help printed materials that can help you to plan your quit attempt and reduce the likelihood of relapse. Many Quitlines also offer free trials of nicotine-replacement products.

A number of published scientific studies have found that telephone Quitlines that employ call-back counseling can be very effective in helping smokers quit. In fact, the more counseling smokers receive from a Quitline, the greater are their chances of being successful in quitting smoking.[22–24]

All callers to the American Cancer Society Quitline receive a follow-up call at 3, 6, and 12 months to evaluate the effectiveness of the program. Smokers can get help finding a Quitline phone counseling program in their area by calling the American Cancer Society at 1–800-ACS-2345 (1–800-227–2345).

Now let's talk about the various methods of addressing the physical addiction of smoking and the best ways to use them from the American Cancer Society's booklet, *Guide to Quitting Smoking.*[15]

Nicotine patches provide a measured dose of nicotine through the skin. You are weaned off the nicotine as you switch to lower-dose nicotine patches over a course of several weeks. Patches can be bought with and without a prescription.

The 16-hour patch works well if you're a light to average smoker (10 or fewer cigarettes per day). It is less likely to cause side effects than are other more long-lasting patches, but it doesn't deliver nicotine at night. So it's not helpful for early-morning withdrawal symptoms, which trouble many smokers.

The 24-hour patch provides a steady dose of nicotine throughout the day and night and helps with early-morning withdrawal. It's often prescribed for heavy smokers (one pack a day or more) but also may cause more side effects. Patches also come in several doses of nicotine. Most smokers should start using a full-strength patch (15 to 22 mg of nicotine) daily for 4 weeks and then use a weaker patch (5 to 14 mg of nicotine) for another 4 weeks. Possible side effects of the nicotine skin patch include

- Redness and itching of the skin
- Dizziness
- Racing heartbeat
- Sleep problems or vivid dreams
- Headache
- Nausea
- Vomiting
- Muscle aches and stiffness

If you experience any of these side effects, you can try a different brand of patch or reduce the amount of nicotine by using a lower-dose patch. Sleep problems also may be short term and may disappear within 3 to 4 days. If side effects are persistent, you also can use another type of nicotine-replacement therapy, such as nicotine gum, nasal spray, or lozenges.

Nicotine gum is a fast-acting form of replacement therapy that comes in 2- or 4-mg strengths. For best results, chew the gum slowly until you notice a peppery taste. Then "park" the gum against your cheek, chewing it and parking it on and off for about 20 to 30 minutes. Avoid acidic foods and drinks such as coffee, juices, and soft drinks for at least 15 minutes before and during gum use. Some cautions for gum use:

- Don't chew more than 20 pieces per day.
- Use the gum for 1 to 3 months and definitely not more than 6 months.
- Use the gum on a fixed schedule for the best results; a schedule of one to two pieces per hour is common.

Side effects can include

- Bad taste
- Throat irritation
- Mouth sores
- Hiccups
- Nausea
- Jaw discomfort
- Racing heartbeat

Stomach and jaw symptoms often result when you use the gum improperly—swallowing it or chewing it too fast. Nicotine gum usually is recommended for 1 to 3 months, with the maximum being 6 months. Tapering the amount of gum chewed may help you to stop using it. But a significant number of people—15% to 20% of those who use this therapy—chew the gum for a year or more. Consult your healthcare provider if you are having trouble stopping smoking after chewing nicotine gum for 6 months.

Nicotine sprays are another popular nicotine-replacement product. They work quickly and relieve withdrawal symptoms very effectively. Most smokers like the nasal spray because it is so effective in relieving cravings and is easy to use. People with allergies or asthma may find that nicotine nasal sprays exacerbate these conditions. The U.S. Food and Drug Administration (FDA) recommends that the spray be prescribed for 3-month periods and that it not be used for longer than 6 months.
Side effects can include

- Nasal irritation
- Runny nose

- Watery eyes
- Sneezing
- Throat irritation
- Coughing

Of all nicotine replacement products, **nicotine inhalers** come closest to mimicking the experience of smoking a cigarette. When you use an inhaler, you activate a cartridge that pushes a nicotine vapor into your mouth. Nicotine inhalers are expensive, and the recommended dose is between 6 and 16 cartridges a day for up to 6 months. Possible side effects are fewer with the nicotine inhaler than with other replacement therapies and tend to occur during the first few days of use. They include

- Coughing
- Throat irritation
- Upset stomach

Nicotine lozenges are the newest type of nicotine-replacement therapy available. They're found in two strengths: 2 and 4 mg. The lozenge manufacturer recommends that they be used as part of a 12-week program. Most people use one lozenge every 1 to 2 hours for 6 weeks, then one lozenge every 2 to 4 hours for weeks 7 to 9, and then one lozenge every 4 to 8 hours for weeks 10 to 12. You shouldn't use more than five lozenges in 6 hours or more than 20 per day. Possible side effects include

- Trouble sleeping
- Nausea
- Hiccups
- Coughing
- Heartburn
- Headache
- Flatulence

When choosing a nicotine-replacement therapy and deciding which is right for you, consider these facts

- Nicotine gums, lozenges, and inhalers allow *you* to control your dosage most effectively; you can use them when your cravings are strongest.
- Nicotine patches need to be applied only once per day.
- Nicotine nasal spray and inhalers work quickly and mimic the sensation of smoking.

- Both inhalers and nasal sprays require a doctor's prescription.
- Using the nicotine patch along with shorter-acting products such as the gum, lozenges, nasal spray, or inhaler is another method of nicotine-replacement therapy. The idea is to get a steady dose of nicotine with the patch and to use one of the shorter-acting products when you have strong cravings.[15]

There are also medications that have been used to help smokers quit, but recently, questions have arisen about their safety. Bupropion (Zyban) is a prescription antidepressant that decreases the symptoms of nicotine withdrawal. It doesn't contain nicotine. Bupropion also tends to cut down on the weight gain that comes with quitting smoking. It shouldn't be taken if you're using alcohol heavily, if you've had a serious head injury, if you've been diagnosed with bipolar disorder, anorexia, or bulimia, or if you've ever had seizures. For heavy smokers, using bupropion with nicotine-replacement therapy is often effective.

Another drug, Chantix (varenicline), also has been approved to help smokers quit. Studies have shown it to be a useful tool in the effort to help smokers quit. However, at the time of publication of this book, the FDA announced that it is requiring manufacturers of both Chantix and Zyban to place a "boxed warning" on the prescribing information for these drugs. The warning will highlight the risk of serious mental health events in users of the drugs, such as depression, hostility, and suicidal thoughts. Patients should contact their health providers immediately if they experience any mood changes when on these drugs. "The risk of serious adverse events while taking these products must be weighed against the significant health benefits of quitting smoking," noted Janet Woodcock, MD, director of the FDA's Center for Drug Evaluation and Research in a press release. "Smoking is the leading cause of preventable disease, disability, and death in the United States, and we know these products are effective aids in helping people quit." According to the FDA, the agency's request for additional boxed warnings on Chantix and Zyban were based on a review of reports to the agency's Adverse Event Reporting System, as well as an analysis of data from clinical trials and the scientific literature

Complementary Therapies for Quitting Smoking

Some people also try **hypnotherapy** or **hypnosis** for quitting smoking. In hypnotherapy, the smoker goes into a trancelike state, during which a therapist may make suggestions that help the smoker quit. The therapist also may suggest that the smoker's feelings of worry, anxiety, and irritability—the side effects of quitting—may decrease.[10]

Hypnosis is considered a complementary medicine therapy, and evidence of effectiveness is not as strong as for the conventional approaches described earlier. According to proponents, hypnosis works best when the therapist can "reframe" the smoker's beliefs about smoking. Many smokers believe that they cannot quit smoking, and the therapist may help them to believe that they can change their behavior. If you do seek out hypnosis, make sure that it is from a licensed clinician or psychologist.[10,15]

Other complementary approaches to quitting smoking include acupuncture. Usually, acupuncture needles are applied to the smoker's ears in this therapy. Some studies suggest that acupuncture may lower the desire to smoke, but there is no solid scientific evidence that it works to help people stop smoking—or remain "smoke-free." For more information on quitting smoking, see the *American Cancer Society Guide to Quitting Smoking*. Available at www.cancer.org/docroot/PED/content/PED_10_13X_Guide_for_Quitting_Smoking.asp.

For more information on how to quit or for counseling or programs that will help you to quit, try these organizations:

- American Cancer Society, 800-ACS-2345, www.cancer.org
- American Lung Association, 1–800-LUNG-USA, www.lungusa.org
- Nicotine Anonymous, 1–877-879–6422, www.nicotine-anonymous.org
- Smokefree.gov, 1–800-QUITNOW, www.smokefree.gov

The Dangers of Smokeless Tobacco

Smokeless tobacco is snuff, chewing tobacco, or a combination thereof. Chewing tobacco comes in the form of long strands of tobacco that are placed between the cheek and gum or teeth. Nicotine is absorbed through the mouth tissues. Snuff is finely ground tobacco packaged in cans or pouches. It is sold in dry and moist forms. Moist snuff—available in small teabag-like pouches—is placed between the lower lip or cheek and gum, and the nicotine is absorbed into the tissues of the mouth. Dry snuff is a powder that is inhaled into the nose. Another new smokeless tobacco product is *snus*—a form of moist snuff made in Sweden and Norway that is produced from air-cured tobacco, water, salt, and flavor additives. Although snus has less tobacco-specific nitrosamines (which can cause cancer) than most other smokeless tobacco products, it still has the potential to cause cancer and a tobacco addiction.

Smokeless tobacco is often marketed by tobacco companies as a way for smokers to use tobacco in smoke-free workplaces, restaurants, and other public places. However, the truth is that these products can lead to oral and pancreatic cancer, addiction to tobacco, receding gums and bone loss around the roots of the teeth, and abrasion and staining of teeth.[25] Smokeless tobacco also may play a role in heart disease and high blood pressure.

Using smokeless tobacco products is also not a good way to quit smoking. Although tobacco companies sometimes imply that smoke-less tobacco products can help you to quit smoking, there is actually no sound evidence to support these claims. Smokers who postpone quitting by using smokeless tobacco or oral tobacco products to get a nicotine fix while in smoke-free settings do not decrease their lung cancer risk. Why? Because they're often still smoking cigarettes, pipes, or cigars in places where smoking is allowed. So they're still at risk for developing all the health conditions associated with smoking, including lung cancer, heart disease, and emphysema.

Quitting Smokeless Tobacco

Quitting smokeless tobacco is not easy, but it can be done.[25] When smoke-less tobacco users try to quit, they may suffer withdrawal symptoms similar to those experienced by smokers. In one Swedish study, oral snuff users reported having as much trouble giving up tobacco as those who used cigarettes.

There are some good reasons to quit using smokeless tobacco. Besides the health risks associated with its use, a smokeless tobacco habit is expensive and carries a social stigma. Bad breath, gum disease, and discolored teeth are very unappealing, especially to dating partners. The spitting required by most smokeless tobacco also can be offensive to many people.

Surveys show that most people who use snuff or chew tobacco would like to quit. In many ways, quitting smokeless tobacco is a lot like quitting smoking. It involves dealing with the physical and psychological aspects of addiction. But there are some aspects of quitting that are unique to smokeless tobacco users. They include

- There is often a stronger need for oral substitutes (having something in the mouth) to take the place of the chew, snuff, or pouch. So some types of nicotine-replacement therapies— namely, nicotine gum and lozenges—may be more effective than others for helping smokeless tobacco users quit. Nicotine gum or lozenges provide an oral substitute for the tobacco chew or snuff. Smokeless tobacco users also can try chewing sugarless candy, sugarless gum, or carrot sticks to deal with oral cravings.

- Heavy users of smokeless tobacco may need higher doses of the nicotine patch to reduce withdrawal symptoms.
- Although bupropion is approved by the FDA for quitting smoking, it's not clear if it's helpful for smokeless tobacco users. A 2007 study found that this medicine helped to reduce cravings and weight gain in people who were trying to quit smokeless tobacco. But those who took bupropion were no more successful in quitting than those who took a placebo (or "sugar pill").
- There are some very visible benefits to quitting smokeless tobacco. The disappearance of mouth sores and gum problems is a readily visible indication of the benefits of quitting, as are the benefits to one's overall health—including reduced risk for heart disease and cancer!

A Word About Some New Nicotine and Tobacco Products

Several new tobacco-containing products and products with nicotine have appeared on the US market in the past few years.[25] However, most are not regulated by the FDA, and although some may be helpful, none has been proven to be effective in helping to quit tobacco use. Some also pose dangers to those who use them.

These products include

- *Nontobacco snuff products.* Packaged like moist snuff in a tin, they contain plants or herbs and sometimes have added flavoring. They are generally considered safe but are not regulated by the FDA. No studies have been done to find out if they are effective in helping people to quit smokeless tobacco.

- *Tobacco lozenges and pouches.* Lozenges and small pouches containing tobacco are now being marketed as ways for smokers to get the effects of tobacco in places where smoking is not permitted. The FDA considers these products as types of smokeless

> tobacco—not aids to quit smoking or products that help to wean the user off tobacco. There is no reason to think that they have fewer health risks than other types of smokeless tobacco.
>
> - *Nicotine lollipops, lip balms, and wafers.* These products contain nicotine, sometimes with sweeteners. Nicotine lollipops (which have been made by some pharmacies in the past) and nicotine lip balms are illegal. Nicotine lollipops pose a special risk to children because they may be mistaken for candy and accidentally eaten. Nicotine wafers also are not safe and are not a good way to quit smoking.

For more on smokeless tobacco, see the American Cancer Society's publication "Smokeless Tobacco and How to Quit," available on their Web site at www.cancer.org.

Smoking in Films

Since the US Surgeon General declared that tobacco was hazardous to health in 1964, education efforts about the dangers of smoking have proliferated, as have smoke-free workplaces, restaurants, and even hotels. Advertising for tobacco has been prohibited on television and radio. Despite these advertising bans, portrayal of tobacco use in movies continues to influence teens to pick up the tobacco habit.

In 1989, the US Congress held hearings after revelations that Philip Morris paid to place Marlboros in the film *Superman II.* The industry amended its voluntary advertising code in 1990 to prohibit paid brand placement of tobacco products in movies. However, tobacco researcher Stanton Glantz, PhD, calls this voluntary code "ineffectual."

In 1998, the tobacco industry signed the Master Settlement Agreement with state attorneys general, which prohibited direct and indirect cigarette advertising to youth and paid product placement in movies. Yet, despite these agreements, the amount of smoking in movies increased rapidly in the 1990s compared with the 1980s. In 2002, the level of smoking in movies was comparable with that observed in 1950, according to a review study published in *Pediatrics* in 2005.[26] And studies of adolescents show that portraying smoking in the movies has a definite effect on teens' attitudes. Those who view images of smoking in the movies are more likely to view smoking as a reflection of everyday life, perceive smoking as an acceptable way to relieve stress, express a nonchalant attitude about smoking in the movies, and although they acknowledge the health risks associated with smoking, find smoking desirable. The more images of smoking that children and teens see in movies, the more likely they are to smoke, according to Glantz.

For smokers, exposure to movie smoking increases their desire to smoke, likelihood to smoke in the future, and perceived positive images of smoking. Exposure to smoking in movies also makes nonsmokers more willing to become friends with a smoker and increases their likelihood of smoking, according to recent research.

If you doubt that smoking in movies has real influence, consider this: A national study of 6522 adolescents aged 10 to 14 years found that those who had the most exposure to smoking in the movies were almost three times as likely to start smoking compared with those who had the lowest exposure. Glantz maintains a Web site, www.smokefree-movies.ucsf.edu, that documents the prevalence of smoking in today's top-grossing movies. On any given week, several of the 10 top-grossing movies are likely to include scenes of smoking, and only half of these movies or fewer portray negative consequences from smoking, Glantz says. Glantz is campaigning for the US film industry to substantially reduce the impact of smoking in the movies on adolescents by taking four steps.

- Rate all newly produced movies that include smoking as "R."
- Post a certificate in the closing credits of every movie saying that no one in the production received anything of value in return for portraying smoking.
- Require that studios and theaters run strong antismoking ads before any film with a tobacco presence.
- Stop identifying tobacco brands in movies. There should be no tobacco brand identification in a movie or even in the background of any scene (such as on a billboard).

"There is a longstanding historical connection between Hollywood and tobacco companies, and that hasn't come to an end," Glantz said in an interview. "Or Hollywood may just be in the grip of inertia," he says. "The problem is that they are perpetuating the positive image of smoking in their films, and research shows this has a real effect on young adults. That's why we're campaigning hard against smoking in the movies."

References

1. National Institute on Drug Abuse. *Research Report: Tobacco Addiction.* NIH Publication 06–4342. Bethesda, MD: NIH; July 2006.

2. National Cancer Institute. *Cigarette Smoking and Cancer: Questions and Answers.* Available at www.cancer.gov/cancertopics/factsheet/tobacco/cancer. Accessed July 19, 2009.

3. American Cancer Society. *Questions About Smoking, Tobacco and Health.* Available at www.cancer.org/docroot/PED/content/PED_10_2x_Questions_About_Smoking_Tobacco_and_Health.asp. Accessed July 19, 2009.

4. American Lung Association. *Tobacco Policy Trend Report. Helping Smokers Quit.* Available at www.lungusa.org/atf/cf/%7B7A8D42C2-FCCA-4604–8ADE-7F5D5E762256%7D/HELPING%20SMOKERS%20QUIT%20-%20STATE%20CESSATION%20COVERAGE%2011–13-08.PDF. Accessed July 19, 2009.

5. Walker MS, Vidrine DJ, Gritz ER, et al. Smoking relapse during the first year after treatment for early-stage non-small-cell lung cancer. *Cancer Epidemiol Biomarkers Prev.* 2006;15: 2370–2377.

6. Centers for Disease Control and Prevention. *Smoking and Tobacco Use. Fact Sheet: Secondhand Smoke.* Available at www.cdc.gov/tobacco/data_statistics/Factsheets/secondhandsmoke.htm. Accessed July 19, 2009.

7. Office of Disease Prevention and Health Promotion, U.S. Department of Health and Human Services. *Healthy People 2010: Understanding and Improving Health.* Available at www.healthypeople.gov. Accessed July 19, 2009.

8. American Cancer Society. *When Smokers Quit—The Health Benefits Over Time.* Available at www.cancer.org/docroot/subsite/greatamericans/content/When_Smokers_Quit.asp. Accessed July 19, 2009.

9. American Cancer Society. *Secondhand Smoke.* Available at www.cancer.org/docroot/PED/content/PED_10_2X_Secondhand_Smoke-Clean_Indoor_Air.asp. Accessed July 19, 2009.

10. Boughton B. "Smoking." *Gale Encyclopedia of Medicine.* Detroit; The Gale Group Inc.; 2002.

11. Anthony JC, Warner LA, Kessler RC. Comparative epidemiology of dependence on tobacco, alcohol, controlled substances and inhalants: basic findings from the National Comorbidity Survey. *Exp Clin Psychopharmacol.* 1994;2:244–268.

12. Russell MAH. The nicotine addiction trap: a 40-year sentence for four cigarettes. *Br J Addiction.* 1990;85:293–300.

13. Anczak JD, Nogler RA. Tobacco cessation in primary care: maximizing intervention strategies. *Clin Med Res.* 2003;1:201–216.

14. Schroeder SA. What to do with a patient who smokes? *JAMA.* 2005;294: 482–487.

15. American Cancer Society. *Guide to Quitting Smoking.* Available at www. cancer.org/docroot/PED/content/PED_10_13X_Guide_for_Quitting_Smoking. asp?sitearea=&level=. Accessed July 19, 2009.

16. Moore D, Aveyar P, Connock M, et al. Effectiveness and safety of nicotine replacement therapy assisted reduction to stop smoking: systematic review and meta-analysis. *BMJ.* 2009;338:b1024.

17. Agency for Healthcare Research and Quality, U.S. Preventive Services Task Force. *Counseling and Interventions to Prevent Tobacco Use and Tobac-co-Caused Disease in Adults and Pregnant Women,* April 2009. Available at www.ahrq.gov/clinic/uspstf09/tobacco/tobaccors2.htm. Accessed July 19, 2009.

18. Nides M, Leischow S, Sarna L, et al. Maximizing smoking cessation in clinical practice: pharmacologic and behavioral interventions. *Prev Cardiol.* 2007;10:S23-S30.

19. Ranney L, Melvin C, Lux L, et al. Systemic review: smoking cessation intervention strategies for adults and adults in special populations. *Ann Intern Med.* 2006;145:845–856.

20. American Cancer Society. *Quitting Smoking—Help for Cravings and Tough Situations.* Available at www.cancer.org/docroot/PED/content/ PED_10_13X_Help_for_Cravings.asp Accessed July 19, 2009.

21. National Institutes of Health. *Research Matters. Smokers Band Together and Quit Together,* June 2, 2008. Available at www.nih.gov/research_ matters/june2008/06022008cigarette.htm. Accessed July 19, 2009.

22. Stead LF, Perera R, Lancaster T. A systematic review of interventions for smokers who contact quitlines. *Tobacco Control.* 2007;16:3–8.

23. Anderson CM, Zhu S. Tobacco quitlines: looking back and looking ahead. *Tobacco Control.* 2007;16:Si81-Si86.

24. Zhu S, Stretch V, Balabanis M, et al. Telephone counseling for smoking cessation: effects of single-session and multiple-session interventions. Journal of consulting and *Clin Psychol.* 1996;64:202–211.

25. American Cancer Society. *Smokeless Tobacco and How to Quit.* Available at www.cancer.org/docroot/PED/content/PED_10_13X_Quitting_Smokeless_ Tobacco.asp?sitearea=&level=. Accessed July 19, 2009.

26. Charlesworth A, Glantz S. Smoking in the movies increases adolescent smoking: a review. *Pediatrics.* 2005;116:1516–1528.

7

Guarding Against Cancer: Staying Safe From Infection

Is Cancer Infectious?

Most people who know at least a little about health and cancer risk would answer "No." And although it's true that you can't catch cancer from someone who has the disease, the interrelationship between infection and cancer is a little more complicated than it may seem at first glance. Although most people understand that factors such as smoking, sun exposure, nutrition, and heredity influence one's risk for cancer, it's harder to make the link between infection and cancer. But the truth is that if you have certain infections, you are more *at risk* for certain cancers. Having these infections doesn't mean you'll necessarily get cancer, but it increases your odds for the disease.

These infections are caused by viruses, or small particles that invade the body's cells and reproduce, eventually causing disease. They also may be caused by bacteria, or small organisms or germs that sometimes cause illness and disease. Certain parasites also can increase the risk for some cancers. Although these parasitic infections are not usually acquired in the United States, they can be a concern for people who live in or travel to other parts of the world.[1] Keep in mind, however, that it's not just any infection that can increase your risk for cancer. So don't worry; having a cold or the flu doesn't increase your chance of getting cancer. The viruses and germs known to cause cancer in the United States are a select group. Table 1 provides a look at the main types and the cancers associated with each of them.

It is important to note that these infections only lead to cancer in a small percentage of cases in the United States. And once someone has cancer, it is not infectious. You can't catch breast cancer or colon

Table 1   Viruses or Bacteria Known to Cause Cancer

Virus or Bacterium	Associated Cancers
Epstein-Barr virus	Nasopharyngeal cancer,[a] some forms of non-Hodgkin lymphoma,[b] such as Burkitt lymphoma, and Hodgkin lymphoma,[b] especially when a person is infected with HIV
Helicobacter pylori	Stomach cancer
Hepatitis B virus	Liver cancer
Hepatitis C virus	Liver cancer and possibly some types of Hodgkin lymphoma
Human herpes virus 8 (HHV-8), also called Kaposi sarcoma–associated herpes virus	Kaposi sarcoma, especially when it occurs with HIV; rare blood cancers such as primary effusion lymphoma and Castleman disease; an overgrowth of lymph nodes that acts very much like lymphoma
HIV	Kaposi sarcoma, cervical cancer, non-Hodgkin lymphoma, and Hodgkin lymphoma, as well as a range of other cancers, including anal, liver, and lung cancer; melanoma; oropharyngeal cancer,[c] leukemia, and colorectal and kidney cancer
Human papillomavirus	Cervical cancer and vulvar, vaginal, penile, and anal cancer
Human T-cell leukemia/lymphoma virus	Adult T-cell leukemia/lymphoma

[a]Nasopharyngeal cancer affects the nasopharynx, an area in the back of the nose toward the base of skull. The nasopharynx is a small boxlike chamber that lies just above the soft palate. It is located at the back of the entrance into the nasal passages.
[b]Non-Hodgkin lymphomas are a diverse group of cancers that arise from the lymphocytes, a type of white blood cell. Hodgkin lymphoma, also known as *Hodgkin disease*, is a type of cancer arising in lymph nodes. Lymph nodes are small hollow structures that contain lymphocytes or white blood cells that attack bacteria and viruses. They are clustered throughout the body, including the neck, armpits, abdomen, and groin (where the abdomen joins the thigh).
[c]Oropharyngeal cancer is a cancer that develops in the part of the throat just behind the mouth, called the *oropharynx*. Sometimes this is called *throat cancer*.
Source: From Refs. 1, 2, 3, and 4.

cancer from someone who has it. And although you can catch some of the viruses and bacteria that may lead to cancers by certain types of contact with an infected person, once the cancer develops, it is not infectious.

News on Viruses and Cancer

What do the viruses that lead to cancer have in common? Many of these viral infections are transmitted through sex or by contact with blood that is contaminated with the virus. So the good news is that you can help to protect yourself from getting these viruses in the first place by using safe-sex practices and by taking other precautions, such as practicing good hygiene and following medical recommendations if you are frequently around blood products.

Another piece of good news is that there are now vaccines that can protect against the two types of human papillomavirus (HPV) that can cause the majority of cervical cancers. The vaccines are considered safe and effective, and many scientists believe that they will help to prevent and greatly decrease cases of cervical cancer in future generations.

Vaccination also can protect you from hepatitis B, an infection that can lead to chronic liver disease, cirrhosis, and liver cancer.[1]

Unfortunately, there is no vaccine yet for hepatitis C (HCV), and the prevalence of HCV infection is high in some parts of the world. In the United States, however, the number of new infections each year has been declining since the late 1980s. An estimated 5% to 10% of those with chronic HCV infection go on to develop severe liver damage and an increased risk of liver cancer. Taking precautions—including practicing safe sex and refraining from sharing needles if you inject drugs intravenously—can help to reduce your risk for this virus.

Most of the people who get infections associated with cancer will not go on to develop cancer, but the risk varies depending on the infection and cancer site. For instance, most people who get the Epstein-Barr virus (EBV), which causes mononucleosis, recover completely. It is only in very rare cases that the virus may trigger cancer years after the initial infection.[2] Some of the viruses that cause cancer are also quite rare in the United States, such as the human T-cell leukemia/lymphoma virus (HTLV-1). Although the risk for some cancers in people with human immunodeficiency virus (HIV) infection is quite high, this risk goes down considerably with HIV treatment.[1]

So let's discuss each of these infections—what they are, what symptoms they cause, how to protect yourself against them, and how and when they may turn to cancer.

HCV: A Stubborn Virus

According to a CDC survey conducted between 1999 and 2002, an estimated 3.2 million people in the United States had chronic HCV infection.

Safer Sex: Protecting Yourself From Sexually Transmitted Diseases—and Cancer

Although many of us have heard the precautions about the importance of protecting oneself from sexually transmitted diseases (STDs), including HIV infection, there is less awareness that some of these STDs can increase cancer risk. Here are the important ingredients for avoiding STDs, according to the Centers for Disease Control and Prevention (CDC)[5,6]:

- Have sex only in a relationship where neither partner is having sex with anyone else. Refrain from sex unless you are in a monogamous relationship with a partner who has been tested and who you know is uninfected.[3]

- If you are not in a monogamous relationship, use a latex condom during sex. They help to prevent the spread of most STDs, although they do not always provide complete protection. When used properly, however, latex condoms can reduce the risk of being infected by HIV. If you or your partner is allergic to latex, plastic (polyurethane) condoms can be used.[3,7]

- Sex practices that are risky include vaginal or anal sex without a condom. Condoms used with a lubricant are less likely to break. Use condoms correctly and consistently in order to be protected from STDS.[3]

- You can spread STDs or HIV through oral sex, although the risk is less than unprotected anal or vaginal sex. If you have oral sex and your partner is male, use a latex or plastic condom. If your partner is female, use a latex barrier such as a natural rubber latex sheet, a dental dam, or a cut-open condom that makes a square. Plastic food wrap also can be used.[7]

- Know your HIV status. If you have had more than one sex partner since your last HIV test or have a partner who has had other sex partners since his or her last HIV test, it's important to get tested. Many states offer anonymous testing.

- If you are diagnosed with an STD, tell your sex partners so that they can be informed and seek medical attention.[3]

Precautions for Healthcare Workers

According to the CDC, healthcare workers who work with or near blood or body fluids should take the following precautions:

- Gloves should be worn during contact with these fluids and should be changed after contact with each patient.

- Hands and other parts of the body should be washed immediately after contact with blood or other body fluids.

- Masks, protective eyewear, or face shields, as well as gowns or aprons, should be worn during procedures that are likely to generate splashes of blood or body fluid.

- To prevent needlestick injuries, needles should not be recapped, bent or broken, or removed from syringes by hand. Sharp items, including reusable needles, should be placed in a puncture-resistant container.[8]

It's the leading cause of death from liver disease in the United States and a major reason for liver transplantation in the United States. About 23% of liver cancer cases in North America are due to chronic infection with HCV.[1] However, as stated before, the number of new HCV infections has declined in recent years in the United States.[1]

Although modern science has been able to protect the US population from a variety of viruses, such as polio and smallpox and even hepatitis B virus (HBV) through vaccines, the defeat of HCV has proven elusive. The reason is that HCV is one of a special set of RNA viruses that can easily outmaneuver the immune system, which normally protects us against viruses by disabling and killing them. However, the HCV can evolve or mutate so fast that the immune system is not able to mount an effective response or attack against it.[9,10]

Because it's so difficult for the immune system to overcome the HCV, many infections with the virus become chronic and can lead to cirrhosis or liver failure. HCV is like a silent thief in that infection with this virus is mild in the early stages, causing few symptoms, and is usually recognized only when it has caused significant damage to the liver. The time from the initial infection to significant liver damage can be as long as 20 years or more.[11]

Some people who get HCV infections are able to fight off the virus during the early stages of the infection, usually within 6 months. However, more than 80% of patients can't get rid of the virus and develop a chronic or long-term infection. People with chronic HCV will have the disease all their lives unless they can be treated successfully with antiviral medications.[1,12]

Chronic HCV damages the liver and can lead to potentially fatal disease such as cirrhosis, which increases the risk for liver cancer and liver failure.

How Is the HCV Transmitted?

Blood transfusions accounted for about 10% of all cases of HCV in the 1970s and 1980s. Since the early 1990s, when improved tests for HCV in donated blood became widespread in the United States, the risk has been negligible.[13]

Any direct or indirect contact with infected blood can transmit the HCV. So contact with needles with blood on them (usually shared needles by intravenous drug users), poorly sterilized medical instruments, or contaminated blood spills can put one at risk for being infected with the virus. It's also possible to get the virus by sharing straws while snorting cocaine or if you've had tattoos or body piercings and the needle was poorly sterilized. Mothers with HCV infections can transmit the virus to

Symptoms of HCV

Most people with HCV have few or no symptoms.[14] This is why it can persist for many years or even decades before it is diagnosed. When symptoms occur, they can include

- Fatigue
- Nausea and loss of appetite
- Dark-colored urine
- Muscle soreness
- Stomach pain
- Jaundice (yellowing of the skin and whites of the eyes)

their babies during birth. Although it's unusual to get the virus through sexual contact, it is possible to transmit the virus through sex.[13,14]

There is a test for the HCV that shows if your body has developed antibodies to HCV. Antibodies are particles your immune system makes to fight infection. A positive test means that at some point in your life you were exposed to HCV.[14]

If your HCV antibody test is positive, your doctor will perform a *viral load test* to see if the HCV virus is in your body and how much is present. If this test is positive, you have chronic infection with HCV, and this means that you eventually may have health problems from the virus.[15]

Who Should Get Tested for HCV?

According the US Department of Veterans Affairs,[15] think about testing if you

- Have ever used a needle to inject drugs
- Had a blood transfusion or organ transplant before 1992
- Are a healthcare worker who has had contact with blood in your work
- Have had long-term kidney dialysis
- Were born to a mother who had HCV
- Have had tattoos or body piercings
- Have ever snorted cocaine
- Have liver disease
- Have a history of drinking a lot of alcohol
- Have had an abnormal liver function test
- Have had multiple sex partners

If You Have HCV

When you have chronic HCV, taking medication can slow the progression of the disease and lessen the chances of getting cirrhosis, which increases the risk for liver cancer. The primary treatment for HCV is a medication called *interferon*, usually given in combination with another drug called *ribovirin*, which boosts the immune system.[14]

One of the reasons for the increase in liver cancer cases among those with HCV is that people are living longer than they did in the past. So, in some cases, people with HCV are now living long enough for their infections to become advanced, and their livers have sustained enough damage to cause cancer.

When you have HCV, other stresses on the body can make cirrhosis and thus liver cancer more likely. According to the American Association for the Study of Liver Disease,[16] these include

- Coinfection with a virus such as HIV or another hepatitis virus
- Alcoholism
- Obesity

If you have a chronic HCV infection, there *are* things you can do to reduce the likelihood of getting liver disease or cancer. The CDC notes these steps for maintaining optimal health in people with HCV[17]:

- Avoid alcohol because it can cause additional liver damage.
- See a liver specialist regularly, and follow his or her advice regarding treatment. Check with your doctor before taking any supplements, over-the-counter medicines, or prescription drugs because these have potential to damage the liver.
- Make sure that you are monitored regularly for liver disease.
- Get the HVA and HBV vaccinations to protect yourself from another liver infection.
- Practice a healthy lifestyle, including nutritious meals, exercise, and avoiding illegal drugs.
- Consider joining an HCV support group, where you can find information about your infection. Your local American Liver Foundation may be able to refer you to a support group.

HBV and Liver Cancer

In 2006, chronic HBV infections affected an estimated 800,000 to 1.4 million Americans, according to the CDC.[18,19] Worldwide, chronic HBV affects about 350 million people, according to the CDC.[18,19] However, although most people who are infected with HBV do not develop serious health problems, about 15% to 40% will have serious complications such as cirrhosis, liver failure, or liver cancer during their lifetime.[20] People who don't recover after an HBV infection are said to have a *chronic infection* or are said to be *chronic carriers* of the virus, and they can transmit the virus to others. Only those with chronic infection are at increased risk for liver diseases, cirrhosis, and liver cancer.[21]

HBV is transmitted through contact with infectious blood or body fluids, such as semen and saliva. It can be spread through[18]

- Sex with an infected person
- Injection drug use that involves sharing needles, syringes, or drug preparation equipment
- Birth to an infected mother
- Contact with blood or open sores of an infected person
- Needle sticks or sharp instrument exposures
- Sharing items such as razors or toothbrushes with an infected person

However, HBV is not spread through food or water, sharing eating utensils, hugging, kissing, hand holding, coughing, or sneezing. HBV is a greater problem internationally than it is in the United States. In areas of the world that have high rates of HBV infection, the virus usually is acquired in childhood, when it is most likely to become chronic.[1, 18]

"In countries such as Hong Kong, Thailand, and China, hepatitis B affects as much as one third of the population," says Eduardo Franco, DrPH, James McGill Professor and director of the Division of Cancer and Epidemiology at McGill University Medical Center in Montreal, Canada. However, vaccination programs in some countries such as Taiwan have helped to decrease the number of HBV infections and resulting liver disease. In fact, a study of a national vaccination program launched in Taiwan more than 20 years ago, published in *Epidemiologic Reviews* in 2006, revealed a 68% decline in deaths from HBV among infants. There also has been a 75% decrease in cases of HBV among children aged 6 to 9 years.[22] In some developing countries, another important cause of HBV is reuse of syringes or needles on multiple patients without adequate sterilization.[1]

In the United States, infection occurs most often in adolescence and adulthood and is associated with high-risk behaviors such as intravenous drug use and having multiple sex partners. The US blood supply has been screened for the HBV since 1973, so there's virtually no risk of getting the virus through a blood transfusion in this country. A vaccine against HBV has been available since 1982. The vaccine is given in three doses and is recommended for all infants, any child up to age 18 who has not been vaccinated, and adults in high-risk groups, such as those traveling to countries in Asia and Africa where the disease is endemic and healthcare workers, who may be exposed to needle sticks or infected blood in their work. Because of blood screening for HBV and vaccinations for young children against the disease, the incidence of HBV has declined greatly in this country.

"It's incredibly important to have vaccination programs for children to protect against hepatitis B," says Elizabeth Ward, PhD, vice president for surveillance and health policy research at the American Cancer Society (ACS). By 2002, 90% of children in the United States aged 19 to 35 months had received the HBV vaccine. Many states also have laws requiring that middle-school children receive the vaccine if they haven't already been vaccinated. The HBV vaccine is available in the United States through the Vaccines for Children program, which provides vaccinations at no or little cost to low-income and uninsured children through their healthcare providers.[1]

The CDC[23] recommends HBV screening (with the HBV surface antigen blood test) for

- People born in geographic areas where HBV affects more than 2% of the population
- Those in the United States who were not vaccinated as children and whose parents were born in countries where HBV is prevalent
- Injection drug users
- Men who have sex with men
- People with abnormal liver function tests
- People who take medications that suppress their immune system
- Pregnant women
- Infants born to HBV-positive mothers
- Household contracts and sex partners of those infected with HBV
- People infected with HIV
- Healthcare workers who have come into contact with body fluids that may be contaminated, such as those who have needle-stick injuries

If pregnant women have evidence of a current infection, the newborn infant should receive HBV immune globulin (HBIG), a sterilized solution obtained from pooled human blood plasma that contains immunoglobulins (or antibodies) to protect against the infectious agents that cause diseases such as HBV. The newborn also should receive the HBV vaccine within 12 hours of birth. These measures are about 85% effective in preventing infections in newborns of women with HBV.[1]

International Travel, Vaccination, and HBV

Most international travelers have a very low risk of contracting HBV unless they are traveling to regions in Asia and Africa where risk is high or intermediate (defined as areas where the number of HBV carriers is greater than 2%). If you are traveling internationally, you should ask your physician if you should get vaccinated for HBV.

Signs of HBV Infection

Although HBV may cause no or few symptoms initially, especially in children under age 5 and in those with weakened immune systems (such as those with HIV infection or those who have received an organ transplant), symptoms can include

- Jaundice
- Fever
- Fatigue
- Loss of appetite
- Nausea
- Vomiting
- Abdominal pain
- Dark urine
- Clay-colored bowel movements
- Joint pain[18]

Unfortunately, although HBV rates have declined among children in the United States, rates have been rising in the United States among men over age 18 and women over age 40. Some scientists think that the solution may be to vaccinate high-risk individuals, including those who have multiple sex partners, men who have sex with men, and injecting drug users. Public health experts also want to increase vaccination rates among children in medically underserved communities. In these communities, parents may find it difficult to get their children to the doctor because of lack of transportation, poverty, or few healthcare providers available nearby.[1]

HPV: A Cause of Cervical and Other Cancers

There are more than 100 types of HPV, only some of which increase the risk for cancer. Some HPVs cause warts—the medical term for these warts is *papillomas*—and they are benign growths. However, the HPV types that cause common warts that grow on the hands and feet are different from those that cause warts or cancer in the genital area.[24]

Some HPVs are also associated with cancer, especially cervical cancer. HPVs also can play a role in causing vulvar, vaginal, penile, and anal cancer and cancer of the oropharynx, the middle part of the throat.[25]

The HPVs that help to cause cancer, particularly cervical cancer, are called *high-risk HPVs*. Among these, HPV-16 and -18 are the most common types among people with cervical cancer.[26]

Genital HPV is very common and is transmitted sexually. Of the more than 100 types of HPV, about 30 can be transmitted sexually. Most HPV infections occur without any symptoms and go away without any treatment within a year or several years. The body's immune system is able to fight off the virus. However, sometimes high-risk HPV infections persist for many years, and in these cases, they can increase a woman's risk for cervical cancer, as well as increasing risk for some other cancers. Genital HPVs also can cause genital warts.[25]

Although there is no cure for long-term infection with HPV, there are ways to treat the genital warts and abnormal cell growths that HPV sometimes can cause.

Persistent HPV infections with high-risk viruses are the major cause of cervical cancer.[25] In 2009, the American Cancer Society estimated that more than 11,000 women in the United States were diagnosed with cervical cancer, and 4070 died from it.[27] Worldwide, cervical cancer is an even bigger problem, especially in developing countries. Cervical cancer is diagnosed in about half a million women worldwide each year, and a quarter of a million women die from it.[25]

Many sexually active women will acquire an HPV infection sometime in their lifetime. Researchers think that women with HPV infections who eventually get cervical cancer often have other risk factors as well, which make the development of cervical cancer more likely. These risk factors include[1,28,29]

- HIV infection
- Diseases that suppress the immune system
- Immune suppression caused by drugs taken after an organ transplant to prevent rejection of the organ
- Smoking

- Long-term use of oral contraceptives
- Coinfection with the genital herpes virus or the sexually trans-mitted bacterium *Chlamydia trachomatis*
- Multiple pregnancies
- Diets low in fruits and vegetables
- Obesity
- Family history of cervical cancer

Cervical Cancer Screening: The Pap Test and the HPV Test

Diagnoses of cervical cancer and mortality from it have decreased dra-matically in the United States largely because of the wide availability of the Papanicolaou test (also called the *Pap smear* or *Pap test*). In a Pap test, a sample of cells is taken from the cervix and examined for abnor-mal cells that could be precancerous or cancerous—abnormal changes that often are caused by long-standing HPV infection. Performing Pap tests reduces the incidence of cervical cancer because the test can help clinicians to detect precancerous lesions that can be treated before they progress to cancer. The Pap test also helps to detect invasive cervi-cal cancer at an early and treatable stage. **Getting regular Pap tests** is extremely important to prevent cervical cancer from developing and to catch cervical cancer early when it is most treatable.[28] (For more information on screening for cervical cancer, see Chapter 8.) There is also a screening test that can look for HPV infection by finding genes or DNA from HPV in cells of the cervix. The test is not recommended for women younger than 30 years of age because many such women have been infected with HPV, and in most of these cases, the virus will disap-pear. Therefore, in women younger than age 30, getting a positive HPV test result is often only confusing and will not help to screen for cervical cancer.

The HPV test can be used by clinicians to screen women older than age 30 for HPV and is another tool that can be used to screen for cervical cancer—along with the Pap test. If you are older than age 30, talk with your doctor about whether an HPV screening test may be useful for you. Some clinicians also use an HPV test to help decide what course of action to take if a woman of any age has a mildly abnormal Pap test.[30]

Vaccines Against HPV

There ares now two HPV vaccines approved by the US Food and Drug Administration (FDA). Gardasil was approved by the FDA in 2006 and protects against HPV-16 and -18, which have been implicated in 70% of cervical cancer cases. It also protects against HPV-6 and -11, which are linked to 90% of cases of genital warts. Gardasil is given in a series of three injections over a 6-month period. It protects against but does not treat an HPV infection.[24]

Another vaccine, Cervarix, was approved by the FDA in 2009 and also protects against HPV-16 and -18, which cause cervical cancer.

Who should get Gardasil or Cervarix? This question is somewhat controversial. Because these vaccines do not treat HPV infection, and because HPV infection is so common among women who are sexually active, the FDA recommends that the vaccine be given to girls before they begin having sex. By giving it to girls before they start having sex, the vaccine could have the most protective effect. The CDC recommends that the vaccines be given to females aged 11 and 12 years and can be given as young as age 9. The CDC also recommends vaccination for women aged 13 to 26 years who have not been vaccinated.[31]

The American Cancer Society (ACS) developed slightly different recommendations in 2007 for HPV Vaccination. The ACS recommends that an HPV vaccine (Gardasil or Ceravix) be given to girls aged 11 and 12 years and as young as 9, at the discretion of doctors. The ACS also agrees that vaccinations should be given to women aged 13 to 18 years. However, the ACS recommendations found that there was *not enough proof of benefit* to recommend vaccines for women age 19 to 26 years. The reasons?[32]

- In clinical trials, women aged 19 to 26 years who had an average of two to four sexual partners before they got vaccinated got less benefit from the vaccine in terms of reducing the overall incidence of abnormal cervical cell changes compared with younger women.
- The vaccine has not been tested in women who have had more than four sexual partners.
- It is not known if the vaccine is cost-effective in this age group. A recent scientific analysis suggests that the vaccination is not cost-effective in women after age 21.
- In October 2009, the FDA also approved the use of Gardasil in males to prevent genital warts. At this time, the ACS has no recommendation regarding the use of either HPV vaccine in males. But the ACS encourages further studies to find out whether HPV vaccines protect against other cancers, along with cervical cancer.[32]

So, again, Gardasil and Cervarix do not protect against an HPV infection that has already occurred. Nor will they clear a specific HPV virus in women who are already infected. But they can provide protection against some HPV types (6, 11, 16, and 18 for Gardasil and 16 and 18 for Cervarix) as long as a woman hasn't yet been infected with these specific types.

Around the world, HPV vaccines are expected to decrease the incidence of cervical cancer. "In the United States, where a lot of women already get screened for cervical cancer with Pap tests, it will help decrease abnormal Pap test results and the morbidity and anxiety associated with these abnormal results," says Debbie Saslow, PhD, ACS director of breast and gynecologic cancer.

Gardasil has been studied for 6 to 7 years, and so far studies have shown that women who receive the vaccine have immunity (or protection against the viruses) for that length of time, according to Saslow. It's not known definitively, however, how long immunity to the HPV viruses ultimately will last in girls or women who get the vaccines. This is why booster shots someday may be needed by those who get the vaccines—for

---

HIV and Cancer

HIV is the virus that causes acquired immune deficiency syndrome (AIDS). It doesn't cause cancers directly. But it does increase the risk for getting several types of cancer, including those that are linked to HPV and the virus known as *human herpes virus type 8* (HHV-8).[2]

HIV is acquired from intimate contact with semen, vaginal secretions, blood, or breast milk of an HIV-infected person. HIV is known to spread through

- Unprotected sex (oral, vaginal, or anal) with an HIV-infected person

- Injections with needles or injection equipment previously used on an HIV-infected person

- Exposure of infants from mothers with HIV infection before birth or during birth

- Breast-feeding by mothers with HIV

- Transfusion of blood products containing HIV (blood has been tested for the virus since 1985)

- Organ transplants from an HIV-infected person (donors are now tested for HIV)[2]

women to have long-term immunity against the HPV viruses that cause cervical cancer.

HIV is not spread through water, by insects, or by casual contact such as talking, shaking hands, sneezing, or sharing telephones or computers. It cannot be spread by hugging, sharing dishes, or sharing a bathroom or kitchen.

HIV infects and destroys white blood cells of the immune system called *helper T cells*. This weakens the immune system and makes it less able to fight off infections. As a result, other viruses such as HPV can cause abnormal growth of the body's cells.

Many scientists think that the body's immune system is crucial for attacking and destroying newly formed cancers. So a weakened immune system may allow new cancers to survive for a long enough time to become serious, life-threatening tumors.

Just to be clear, HIV infection is not the same as AIDS. AIDS is the most advanced stage in HIV infection, Most people living with HIV infection do not have AIDS. According to the CDC, people with HIV infection are considered to have AIDS if they have a very low count of helper T cells (<200 per µL of blood) and/or they have one or more AIDS-defining illnesses. Most AIDS-defining illnesses are infections that are rare in people with a healthy immune system.

Some forms of cancer are also considered AIDS-defining—Kaposi sarcoma, some types of non-Hodgkin lymphoma, and invasive cervical cancer. People with AIDS and others living with HIV infection who do not have AIDS also are more likely to develop other types of cancers.

Kaposi Sarcoma: What Causes It?

Kaposi sarcoma (KS) is a cancer that develops from the cells that line lymph or blood vessels and causes patches of abnormal tissue to grow under the skin. Kaposi sarcoma's distinctive tumors appear as purple, red, or brown lesions on the skin. The color comes from the fact that they are rich in blood vessels. The cancer is caused by the Kaposi sarcoma herpes virus (KSHV), which is also called *human herpes virus type 8* (HHV-8). Although people do not develop KS without first getting infected with HHV-8, most people who are infected with HHV-8 never develop KS. Someone who is infected with HHV-8 is more likely to develop KS if their immune system doesn't work properly. In people with AIDS, the immune system is compromised, and the KS is caused by an interaction between HIV, the weakened immune system, and HHV-8.

KS is now divided into four main types. One type is called *sporadic* or *classic Kaposi sarcoma*. In comparison with other types of KS, the lesions in this type do not grow as quickly, and new lesions do not develop as often. *Endemic Kaposi sarcoma* is more common in Africa than in other places such as Europe or North America. *Epidemic Kaposi sarcoma* is related to AIDS. Some people—usually organ transplant recipients—get a type of KS that is called *immunosuppression-associated Kaposi sarcoma*.[1]

KS associated with HIV infection and AIDS is the most likely of all four types to involve multiple lesions and the worst prognosis.

Sexual contact is believed to be the major way that people are infected with HHV-8. Yet, in Africa, this infection is seen in children, so scientists think other modes of transmission may be possible.[1]

The incidence of KS peaked among men in the United States aged 20 to 54 years in 1989 and then declined markedly, probably because of changes in sexual practices that reduced the transmission of HIV and HHV-8. In 1996, highly active antiretroviral therapy (HAART), a treatment for AIDS that has helped make this disease a chronic condition rather than a rapidly fatal one in many cases, also decreased the incidence of KS. HAART reduces the risk of KS among people already infected with HIV and also is helpful in treating the tumors of KS.[1]

Protecting against KS means protecting against the viruses that cause it—practicing safe sex, abstaining from injection drug use, or using sterile equipment during usage of intravenously administered drugs.[1]

Other HIV-Related Cancers

Not long after the link between HIV and KS was described, researchers began to notice links with some other forms of cancer. Some of these are considered by the CDC to be AIDS-defining—invasive cervical cancer and some types of non-Hodgkin lymphoma. Several other cancers are also more common in people living with HIV. A 2008 paper in the *Annals of Internal Medicine*[33] updated this research by comparing cancer occurrence in participants from two large ongoing studies of HIV-positive people (a total of more than 54,000 patients) with the overall US population from 1992 to 2003. The researchers concluded that HIV-infected people are at higher risk for KS, anal and vaginal cancer, cervical cancer, non-Hodgkin lymphoma, Hodgkin lymphoma, liver cancer, lung cancer, melanoma, oropharyngeal cancer, leukemia, and colorectal and kidney cancer. The relationship between these cancers and HIV is complex and still not entirely understood, but it's believed that cancers can develop and grow more quickly in those with HIV infection because they have weakened immune systems from the virus. People who have HIV infection should be aware of their increased risk for a range of cancer types and should ask their doctors about screening tests that are available for some of these cancers. They also should discuss treatments that can lower their cancer risk.

EBV and Cancer

EBV is best known for causing infectious mononucleosis, also known as "mono" or the "kissing disease." In addition to kissing, it can be passed from person to person by coughing, sneezing, or sharing drinking or eating utensils. Most people in the United States are infected with EBV before age 20, although not everyone develops the symptoms of mono. The virus remains in the body throughout life, but after the first few weeks of infection, most people never have any other symptoms. Infection with EBV increases a person's risk of getting *nasopharyngeal cancer* (cancer of the area in the back of the nose) and certain types of fast-growing lymphomas such as *Burkitt lymphoma*. It also may be linked to *Hodgkin disease* and some cases of *stomach cancer*. These cancers (except for Hodgkin disease) are more common in Africa and parts of Southeast Asia. Overall, very few people who have been infected with EBV will ever develop these cancers.[1]

For the EBV to cause cancer, usually some other risk factors have to be present as well. The strongest risk factors that can increase the odds for cancer in someone infected with EBV are being infected as a very young child and coinfection with HIV or having AIDS. Other immune-system deficiencies, such as those that affect people who have had organ transplants, also can increase the odds for cancer in those infected with EBV.

There is no practical way to prevent getting the EBV because it is transmitted through contact with saliva and is present in the saliva of most healthy people.[1] However, it is possible to protect against HIV infection through practicing safe sex, refraining from intravenous drug use, and following hygiene practices if you are a healthcare worker.

Helicobacter pylori and Stomach Cancer Risk

Stomach cancer is the fourth most common cancer in the world and is the fifteenth most common cancer in the United States.[1] Infection with the *Helicobacter pylori* (*H. pylori*) bacterium increases the risk of developing stomach cancer to some extent, but how much it increases the risk is still open to question. *H. pylori* infection also causes chronic gastritis and peptic ulcers. According to recent studies, more than 50% of people over age 50 are infected with *H. pylori*. In the United States, the prevalence of *H. pylori* infection tends to increase as people get older.[1]

It's not known with absolute certainty how *H. pylori* is transmitted, but it may spread from person to person by oral-fecal contact or oral-oral contact. Because the mode of infection isn't known definitively, there's really no way to prevent infection. However, experts with the ACS recommend washing hands thoroughly, eating food that has been prepared and stored properly, and drinking water from a clean, safe source.[1]

H. pylori infection can be treated with medications known as *proton pump inhibitors* (PPIs) and two antibiotics. If treatment fails, a combination of a PPI, bismuth salts, and two antibiotics is often tried. This regimen is effective in clearing the infection in 90% of patients. Research on a preventive vaccine is ongoing—although clinical trials of such vaccines so far have been disappointing.[1]

The good news is that stomach cancer is fairly uncommon in the United States. And the vast majority of people who have *H. pylori* in their stomachs never develop cancer. If you do have other risk factors for stomach cancer—such as a history of such cancer in your family—it may be wise to talk with your physician about screening for infection with *H. pylori*. Other risks for stomach cancer include[34]

- Aging
- Diets with large amounts of smoked foods, salted fish and meat, and pickled vegetables and low in fresh fruits and vegetables
- Smoking
- Obesity
- Previous stomach surgery
- Some inherited cancer syndromes such as hereditary nonpolyposis colorectal cancer (HNPCC), also known as *Lynch syndrome* and *familial adenomatous polyposis* (FAP)
- A history of stomach polyps or benign growths

A Rare Virus: HTLV-1

Human T-cell leukemia/lymphoma virus (HTLV-1) is rare in the United States, although it is more common in other areas, such as southern Japan, the Caribbean, Africa, and parts of South America. Like HIV, this virus is spread by sexual intercourse or by injection with contaminated needles and can be transmitted from mother to child during birth and breast-feeding. In the United States, all donated blood is routinely tested for HTLV-1.[2]

The cancer associated with HTLV-1 is a rare type of non-Hodgkin lymphoma called *adult T-cell leukemia/lymphoma.*[2]

References

1. American Cancer Society. *Cancers Linked to Infectious Disease. Cancer Facts and Figures 2005.* Available at www.cancer.org/docroot/STT/content/ STT_1x_Cancer_Facts__Figures_2005.asp. Accessed July 29,2009.

2. American Cancer Society. *Infectious Agents and Cancer.* Available at www.cancer.org/docroot/PED/content/PED_1_3X_Infectious_Agents_and_ Cancer.asp. Accessed July 14, 2009.

3. American Cancer Society. *Detailed Guide: HIV Infection and AIDS.* Available at www.cancer.org/docroot/CRI/CRI_2_3x.asp?dt=78. Accessed July 16, 2009.

4. National Cancer Institute. *Hepatitis C and Lymphoma: Questions and Answers.* Available at www.cancer.gov/newscenter/pressreleases/HepCLymphomaQandA. Accessed July 14, 2008.

5. Centers for Disease Control and Prevention. *HIV and AIDS: Are You at Risk?* Available at www.cdc.gov/hiv/resources/brochures/at-risk.htm. Accessed November 30, 2009.

6. Centers for Disease Control and Prevention. *STDs and Pregnancy—The Facts.* Available at www.cdc.gov/std/pregnancy/the-facts/. Accessed July 14, 2009.

7. Centers for Disease Control and Prevention. *Can I Get HIV from Oral Sex?* Available at www.cdc.gov/hiv/resources/qa/qa19.htm. Accessed July 29, 2009.

8. Centers for Disease Control and Prevention. *Universal Precautions for Prevention of Transmission of HIV and other Bloodborne Infections. Fact Sheet.* Available at www.cdc.gov/ncidod/dhqp/bp_universal_precautions. html. Accessed July 14, 2009.

9. The C. Everett Koop Institute, Dartmouth Medical School. *Hepatitis C: An Epidemic for Anyone. The Facts. Viruses.* Available at www.epidemic.org/ theFacts/viruses/.

10. The C. Everett Koop Institute, Dartmouth Medical School. *Hepatitis C: An Epidemic for Anyone. The Facts. Hepatitis C. The Hepatitis C Virus.* Available at www.epidemic.org/theFacts/hepatitisC/hepatitisC/. Accessed July 14, 2009.

11. The C. Everett Koop Institute, Dartmouth Medical School. *Hepatitis C: An Epidemic for Anyone. The Facts. Hepatitis C: The Silent Epidemic.* Available at www.epidemic.org/theFacts/hepatitisC/silentEpidemic/. Accessed July 14, 2009.

12. The C. Everett Koop Institute, Dartmouth Medical School. *Hepatitis C: An Epidemic for Anyone. The Facts. Hepatitis C. Disease Progression.* Available at www.epidemic.org/theFacts/hepatitisC/diseaseProgression/. Accessed on July 14, 2009.

13. The C. Everett Koop Institute, Dartmouth Medical School. *The Facts. Hepatitis C Transmission.* Available at www.epidemic.org/theFacts/hepatitisC/transmission/. Accessed July 14, 2009.

14. US Department of Veterans Affairs. *Hepatitis C Fact Sheet.* Available at www.hepatitis.va.gov/vahep?page=basics-01-00. Accessed July 14, 2009.

15. US Department of Veterans Affairs. *Hepatitis C: Getting Tested Fact Sheet.* Available at www.hepatitis.va.gov/vahep?page=test-print&pp=pf. Accessed July 14, 2009.

16. Ghany MG, Strader DB, Thomas DL, et al. *American Association for the Study of Liver Disease Guidelines. Diagnosis, Management and Treatment of Hepatitis C: An Update,* 2009. Available at www.aasld.org/practiceguidelines/Documents/Bookmarked%20Practice%20Guidelines/Diagnosis_of_HEP_C_Update.pdf. Accessed July 14, 2009.

17. Centers for Disease Control and Prevention. *Hepatitis C: FAQs for the Public.* Available at www.cdc.gov/hepatitis/C/cFAQ.htm. Accessed July 14, 2009.

18. Centers for Disease Control and Prevention. *Hepatitis B: Frequently Asked Questions.* Available at www.cdc.gov/ncidod/diseases/hepatitis/b/faqb.htm. Accessed July 14, 2009.

19. Centers for Disease Control and Prevention. Recommendations for identification and public health management of persons with chronic hepatitis B virus infection. *MMWR.* 2008;57(RR-8).

20. Lok AS, McMahon BJ. *American Association for the Study of Liver Diseases Guidelines. Chronic Hepatitis B,* 2007. Available at www.aasld.org/practiceguidelines/Documents/Bookmarked%20Practice%20Guidelines/Chronic%20Hepatits%20B.pdf. Accessed July 16, 2009.

21. Centers for Disease Control and Prevention. *The ABCs of Hepatitis Fact Sheet.* Available at www.cdc.gov/hepatitis/Resources/Professionals/PDFs/ABCTable_BW.pdf. Accessed July 14, 2009.

22. Chien YC, Jan CF, Kuo HS, et al. Nationwide hepatitis B vaccination program in Taiwan: effectiveness in the 20 years after it was launched. *Epidemiol Rev.* 2006;28:126–135.

23. Centers for Disease Control and Prevention. *Testing and Public Health Management of Persons with Chronic Hepatitis B Virus Infection.* Available at www.cdc.gov/Hepatitis/HBV/TestingChronic.htm. Accessed July 14, 2009.

24. American Cancer Society. *Human Papilloma Virus, Cancer, and HPV Vaccines—Frequently Asked Questions.* Available at www.cancer.org/docroot/CRI/content/CRI_2_6x_FAQ_HPV_Vaccines.asp. Accessed July 16, 2009.

25. National Cancer Institute. *Human Papillomaviruses and Cancer: Questions and Answers.* Available at www.cancer.gov/cancertopics/factsheet/Risk/HPV. Accessed July 16, 2009.

26. Foerster V, Murtagh J. Human papillomavirus (HPV) vaccines: a Canadian update. In: *Issues in Emerging Health Technologies,* Vol. 109. Ottawa: Canadian Agency for Drugs and Technologies in Health; 2007.

27. American Cancer Society. *Cancer Facts and Figures 2009.* Available at www.cancer.org/docroot/STT/content/STT_1x_Cancer_Facts__Figures_2009.asp?from=fast. Accessed July 16, 2009.

28. American Cancer Society. *Detailed Guide: Cervical Cancer.* Available at www.cancer.org/docroot/CRI/CRI_2_3x.asp?rnav=cridg&dt=8. Accessed July 16, 2009.

29. American Cancer Society. *Cervical Cancer Linked to Birth Control Pills. Fact Sheet,* April 16, 2003. Available at www.cancer.org/docroot/NWS/content/NWS_1_1x_Cervical_Cancer_Linked_To_Birth_Control_Pills.asp. Accessed July 16, 2009.

30. American Cancer Society. *Thinking About Testing for HPV?* Available at www.cancer.org/docroot/CRI/content/CRI_2_6x_Thinking_About_Testing_for_HPV.asp?sitearea=&level=. Accessed July 16, 2009.

31. Centers for Disease Control and Prevention. *HPV Vaccine: Questions and Answers.* Available at www.cdc.gov/vaccines/vpd-vac/hpv/vac-faqs.htm. Accessed July 16, 2009.

32. American Cancer Society. *American Cancer Society Recommendations for Human Papillomavirus (HPV) Use to Prevent Cervical Cancer and Pre-Cancers.* Available at www.cancer.org/docroot/CRI/content/CRI_2_6X_ACS_Recommendations_for_HPV_Vaccine_Use_to_Prevent_Cervical_Cancer_and_Pre-Cancers_8.asp?sitearea=&level=. Accessed July 16, 2009.

33. Patel P, Hanson DL, Sullivan PS. Incidence of types of cancer among HIV-infected persons compared with the general population in the United States, 1992–2003. *Ann Intern Med.* 2008;148:728–736.

34. American Cancer Society. *Detailed Guide—Stomach Cancer. What Are the Risk Factors for Stomach Cancer?* Available at www.cancer.org/docroot/CRI/content/CRI_2_4_2X_What_are_the_risk_factors_for_stomach_cancer_40.asp. Accessed July 16, 2009.

8

Get Screened for Cancer:
Which Tests Are Best?

Although Charlie Kelley was a bit reluctant to go through his first colon-oscopy, he decided to undergo the test in November 2008. His mother had a history of polyps (benign growths) in her colon—growths that some-times can turn cancerous if not removed. So Charlie made the decision to have a colonoscopy at age 40. His physician advised him that he should start colorectal cancer screening 10 years earlier than is recommended for the general population—because of his family history.

"Although I wasn't having any symptoms, and it was just a precaution-ary thing, the test found three polyps, and one was highly active cancer," says Charlie, a musician who lives in Nashville. During his colonoscopy, the gastroenterologist was able to remove all three of the growths, includ-ing the cancerous one, and sent them out for testing. That December, Charlie had surgery that removed 10 inches of his colon to treat his remaining cancer. Luckily, the cancer was at an early stage and highly curable when it was caught. After 6 weeks of recovery, Charlie returned to work with no side effects.

"I'm very positive about having gone through the colonoscopy," Charlie says. "When I told my friends my story, it spurred a few of those over 50 to get the test as well. That's the greatest gift for me out of this whole experience."

Charlie emphasizes that colonoscopies are important because they can catch cancer early, when the chance for cure is improved. "It's poten-tially a lifesaving procedure, and I don't think people should be shy about it," he says.

Charlie Kelley's story illustrates the importance of getting screen-ing tests for cancer. These screening tests include those that screen for breast, colon, and cervical cancer.

These tests are often our best hope for detecting and catching cancer early, when it is most curable. Getting screened regularly and appropriately for cancer is, in fact, an important step for many people in preventing the diagnosis of a late-stage cancer. Although some screening tests are recommended for most people, especially as people grow older, others are meant only for high-risk populations.

In this chapter we'll discuss screening tests for six different kinds of cancer: breast, cervical, colon, prostate, lung, and ovarian. Screening for three of the most common cancers—breast, colon, and cervical—is known to be very effective for early detection. Screening also can help to prevent colon and cervical cancer because it can spot precancerous changes or growths that then can be treated successfully. Although routine screening for prostate, lung, and ovarian cancer isn't recommended, the pros and cons of these tests also merit discussion as well. We'll talk about the scientific evidence concerning the effectiveness of each test in screening for different kinds of cancer, as well as any controversies surrounding each test.

Mammograms for Breast Cancer: A Necessary Choice

Mammograms remain the "gold standard" for detecting breast cancer. Clinical trials have found that women who get mammograms are less likely to die of breast cancer than those who do not—and it's the only breast screening test that has been proven to reduce mortality from this disease, according to Therese Bevers, MD, medical director of the Cancer Prevention Center and associate professor at the University of Texas MD Anderson Cancer Center.

The overall technical quality of mammograms also has improved over the years. With this greater resolution, mammograms allow radiologists to be much more precise in pinpointing tumors. Mammograms aren't perfect—they can miss some cancers and sometimes indicate a problem where none exists—but they are still one of the best tools we have for screening for breast cancer.[1,2] Death rates from breast cancer in the United States have been declining since the 1990s, and one reason is early detection by mammography screening, as well as improvements in treatment.[2]

Breast cancers found by screening exams such as mammograms tend to be smaller and are more likely to be confined to the breast. Those that are felt by touch, by contrast, tend to be larger and more likely to have spread beyond the breast. The size of a breast cancer and how far it has spread are important factors in predicting the survival outlook for a woman with this disease. This is why mammograms are so important: This test can find cancers before they start to cause symptoms. Most scientists and physicians agree that mammograms save thousands of lives each year, and more could be saved if more women took advantage of these tests.[1]

However, mammograms tend to be more reliable in women 50 years of age and older than they are in women aged 40 to 49 years. And because breast cancer is more common among women older than age 50, the benefit of mammography is greater than it is for younger women. In fact, there's been a debate among doctors and scientists about what should be the best recommendation regarding screening mammograms for women aged 40 to 49 years. The American Cancer Society and the American College of Radiology recommend yearly mammograms for women aged 40 to 49 years, whereas the National Cancer Institute and the American College of Obstetricians and Gynecologists recommend screening mammograms every 1 to 2 years for this age group. In November 2009, the US Preventive Services task force recommended against *routine* mammography for average-risk women in this age group, but they suggested that women speak with their physician regarding the best time to begin mammography every 2 years.[3,4]

Screening mammograms for women aged 40 to 49 years may be more likely than those for women aged 50 years and older to indicate cancer might be present where none exists. Some scientific studies have shown that this type of false-positive result can occur in up to half the women in this age group if they receive annual mammograms between the ages of 40 and 49 years, whereas other studies have shown no difference in the false-positive rate between different age groups. A false-positive test result can result in increased anxiety for a woman, as well as unnecessary procedures (usually additional mammograms, ultrasound, or other imaging tests but less often a biopsy).[3,4]

The results of individual studies vary, but the summary of studies looking at lives saved among women aged 40 to 49 years shows a survival advantage for women in this age group who have mammograms regularly. The debate currently involves whether the benefit of screening in this age group is much less than in older women or if it is slightly less and whether that benefit outweighs the nonmonetary costs (such as false-positive results, additional mammograms, etc.). Experts in cancer screening have reached very different answers to these questions because they have different views of a number of technical points, such as which studies should be included in the summaries and how to adjust for imperfections in studies conducted several decades ago. For ethical reasons, there will never be another clinical study that randomly assigns some women to screening mammograms and tells others not to have mammograms. Therefore, it seems unlikely that there will ever be an unequivocal answer to this question.

Given this controversial state of affairs, it is important for women in this age group to have an informed discussion with their healthcare providers about the costs and benefits of mammography before age 50. Looking toward the future, most breast cancer researchers are confident that a more complete understanding of this disease and advances in technology will improve the accuracy of early detection of breast cancer so that more lives can be saved with fewer side effects.[3,4] While the American Cancer Society recommends yearly mammograms for women at average risk for breast cancer aged 40 years and older, its recommendations for women at above-average risk are somewhat different. These screening guidelines say[5,6]

- Women at high risk (>20% lifetime risk) should get a magnetic resonance imaging (MRI) screening and a mammogram every year. For most women at high risk, screening with MRI and mammograms should begin at age 30 and continue for as long as the woman is in good health. Yet, because the evidence is limited regarding the best age at which to start screening, this decision should be based on shared decision making between patients and their healthcare providers.
- Women at moderately increased risk (15% to 20% lifetime risk) should talk with their doctors about the benefits and limitation of adding MRI screening to their yearly mammogram.
- Yearly MRI screening is not recommended for women whose lifetime risk of breast cancer is less than 15%.

(For more on MRI screening for breast cancer and for those women at high risk, see page 131.)

A mammogram is an X-ray of the breast; a conventional mammogram produces a black-and-white image of the breast tissue on a large sheet of film. It's also possible today to be screened by **digital mammography.** This test uses an electronic process to collect and display X-ray images on a computer screen. This allows radiologists to lighten or darken the image before it is printed on film. Images also can be manipulated by the radiologist to magnify or zoom in on an area. One large clinical trial of 49,000 women screened with both digital and film mammograms (called the Digital Mammographic Screening Trial) found that digital mammograms can be better than regular mammograms for women under age 50, those who have not gone through menopause, and those with dense breasts.[7-9] However, digital mammogram machines are more expensive than traditional film mammogram machines and not yet available in some communities.

Yet, whether or not you undergo a digital or regular mammogram, it's important that you get this test regularly, especially if you are over age 50. The American Cancer Society and The American College of Radiology recommend that women aged 50 years and older (like those between 40 and 49 years of age) should have a screening mammogram every year and should continue to do so for as long as they are in good health. The National Cancer Institute and the American College of Obstetricians and Gynecologists also recommend annual mammograms for women 50 years of age and older (as well as mammograms every 1–2 years from ages 40–49). The US Preventive Services Task Force recommends mammography every 2 years for women aged 50 to 74 years and concludes that there is not enough evidence to recommend for or against mammography for women aged 75 years and older (or 40 to 49 years).[3,4]

Recent studies indicate that many women are not screened often enough, according to the American Cancer Society. Overall, about half of women over age 40 have had a mammogram within the past year, and about two-thirds have had one within the past 2 years. But only about 40% of women with less than a high school education, 24% of uninsured women, 38% of Asian Americans, and 35% of recent (<10 years) immigrants have been screened in the past year. Many women also don't have access to this important screening tool.[2] To find low-cost mammograms in their area, women can call the American Cancer Society at 1–800-ACS-2345.

Mammograms are not fun—having your breasts squeezed between two plates of plastic is very uncomfortable. But I've always been happy to put up with the discomfort and inconvenience. Why? I'm comforted by the idea that mammograms are available to me—and that this technology can detect cancers at a stage when they are less likely to spread. Having a regular yearly mammogram is one step I can take to be proactive about my breast health and to catch cancer early, before it can become deadly, if I, like my mother did, ever do get breast cancer.

Besides mammograms, there are other tests for breast cancer, and they can be beneficial for certain women. What are these tests for breast cancer, and who can benefit from them?

MRI uses magnetic fields to produce detailed cross-sectional images of tissue structures. Scientific studies have shown that MRI is a good screening tool for some women who have an increased risk for breast cancer—usually those who have a significant family history or a genetic mutation—and often can find cancers that are missed on mammograms. At the same time, MRI occasionally can miss cancers that mammography would detect, and it is a more expensive screening method. And an MRI is significantly more likely than a mammogram to indicate a cancer where none exists. So MRI is not recommended for those who have an average risk or even a slightly elevated risk for breast cancer. After reviewing scientific evidence about MRI and its benefits, a panel of experts from the American Cancer Society[5] recommended screening MRI for

- Women with a *BRCA* mutation
- A first-degree relative of someone with a *BRCA* mutation but who is untested
- Women with a lifetime breast cancer risk of 20% to 25% or greater, usually from a strong family history, sometimes combined with other risk factors
- Women who have had radiation to the chest (usually to treat Hodgkin disease) between the ages of 10 and 30 years, which increases the risk for breast cancer later in life
- Patients or their first-degree relatives with Li-Fraumeni syndrome, Cowden syndrome, and Bannayan-Riley-Ruvalcaba syndromes—All these genetic syndromes confer a greatly increased risk of breast cancer.

The panel also found that there was insufficient scientific evidence either for or against MRI screening for women who fall into the following groups:

- Having a lifetime breast cancer risk of 15% to 20%
- Having a past diagnosis of lobular carcinoma in situ or atypical lobular hyperplasia—two conditions marked by changes or abnormal cells in the lobules, the parts of the breast that produce milk (Lobular carcinoma in situ and atypical lobular hyperplasia are not breast cancer, but they increase the risk for developing the disease.)
- A past diagnosis of atypical ductal hyperplasia—a condition in which cells that line the milk ducts of the breast grow abnormally (It is not cancer, but it can indicate an increased cancer risk for some women.)
- Extremely dense breasts on mammography
- Women with a personal history of breast cancer, including ductal carcinoma in situ

The panel recommended against MRI screening for

- Women with less than a lifetime risk of 15% for breast cancer

So what if you fall into one of the groups for which the benefits of MRI are not clear? The obvious choice—especially if you have a previous history of cancer—is to talk with your clinician about what kinds of tests are best for you.

One question I had after I read the American Cancer Society panel's report: How can one assess one's risk for breast cancer? In other words, did I fall into one of the risk groups that would benefit from MRI? Risk of breast cancer can be assessed by a genetic counselor using a mathematical model known as BRCAPRO or the Breast and Ovarian Analyses of Disease Incidence and Carrier Estimation Algorithm (BOADICEA). Some genetic counselors use mathematical models known as the Gail, Claus, or Tyrer-Cusick models, along with considering the family history of breast cancer and personal history of the disease.

If you fall into the 20% and above risk group because of a family history of the disease, you probably would benefit from a visit with a genetic counselor, who can assess you for a possible genetic mutation. To find a genetic counselor near you, you can inquire through your health plan or log onto the Cancer Genetics Services Directory of the National Cancer Institute at www.cancer.gov/search/geneticsservices/.

Another way to assess one's cancer risk is to use an online risk assessment tool (see Chapter 2), available through the National Cancer Institute's Web site at www.cancer.gov/bcrisktool/ or at www.breastcancerprevention.org. However, there are important cautions for using these tools. They were devised with the Gail model, which considers history of breast cancer only in first-degree relatives (mother, sister, or daughter) as a risk factor. Cases of breast cancer in second-degree relatives (such as an aunt or cousins), which could indicate a strong family history of the disease, do not factor into the tools' risk calculation. If you do have a strong history of breast cancer in second- or first-degree relatives, it may be wise to get more information from your clinician and a genetic counselor.

When I used the online tool at www.breastcancerprevention.org, I answered a few questions about my age (51), my reproductive history, and my family history. The test showed that my risk for developing breast cancer up to age 80 was 13%, even with my family history of breast cancer. In comparison, the average risk of a woman aged 50 years with no risk factors is 5% by age 80, according to the tool. So, although my risk is clearly elevated, MRI would not be the best screening tool for me.

Breast ultrasound is usually used to evaluate an abnormality found on a mammogram or during a clinical exam. It uses sound waves to produce images of structures within the body. Breast ultrasound can help to tell if an area or growth within the breast is a cyst or solid tissue. A cyst is a fluid-filled sac or pouch that is usually a benign growth. In cases in which the ultrasound finds solid tissue, a biopsy would be needed to determine if the solid growth is cancerous. Biopsy is usually not employed for screening in people without symptoms because it does not consistently detect early signs of breast cancer, such as microcalcifications. Microcalcifications are tiny deposits of calcium in the breast that may indicate that cancer is present.[8]

Tools for Finding Breast Cancer:
Clinical Breast Exam and Self-Awareness

Aside from screening tests such as a mammogram, every woman should have a **clinical breast exam** by a clinician to look for signs of breast cancer. The American Cancer Society recommends that women in their 20s should have this exam at least every 3 years and should start annual exams at age 40. During a clinical breast exam, a doctor or nurse will thoroughly examine your breasts for any lumps or suspicious areas and will feel the texture and size of any abnormalities. During an exam, the clinician also will note any changes in the nipples or skin of your breasts. The lymph nodes under the armpit and above the collarbones will be palpated (or felt) to determine any enlargement or firmness that could signal cancer.[10]

Although monthly **breast self-exam** (BSE) used to be emphasized as a way for women to note changes in their breasts and to find breast cancer, many experts now recommend **self-awareness** instead. The reason is that scientific studies haven't shown a real benefit to teaching a specific technique for monthly BSE to detect breast cancer, according to Bevers. However, that said, if a woman does want to do BSE, it's best to ask your doctor or nurse how to do it properly.

Even without doing BSE, women should be aware of how their breast look and feel normally. They should note any changes in the feel of their breast, such as a lump or an irritation, and any changes in the way the breasts look, such as dimpling, nipple retraction (the nipple turning inward), redness, scaliness, or thickness of the nipple or breast skin. Finally, any breast or nipple pain or a discharge other than breast milk should be reported to your doctor.

Women should watch not just for lumps but also for other changes in the way their breasts look and feel. Some breast cancers are marked by symptoms other than lumps. For instance, the rare condition known as *inflammatory breast cancer* is marked by redness, skin thickening, warmth, and swelling.[1]

"Most people touch their bodies—including their breasts—without thinking about it," Bevers says. "And what we've found is that being aware of the changes in your body can be just as good or better at finding a breast cancer as breast self-exam. It's rare that a woman will come in and say to me: 'I found a lump while doing a breast self-exam.' It's more often: 'My husband felt it or I discovered it while dressing or showering.'"

That said, women should take care to feel and note changes in the entire breast. If you feel that you need direction on how to examine your breasts, you also can find instructions on how to do a BSE at the American Cancer Society's' Web site at www.cancer.org/docroot/CRI/content/CRI_2_6x_How_to_perform_a_breast_self_exam_5.asp. And don't hesitate to ask your doctor or nurse any questions you may have about BSE.

Cervical Cancer: Screening Saves Lives

The American Cancer Society estimates that in 2009, 11,270 cases of invasive cervical cancer will be diagnosed in the United States, and 4,070 women will die from the disease.[11] More than 50% of women who are diagnosed with invasive cervical cancer have not undergone screening with the **Papanicolaou (Pap) test**.[12]

Fortunately for many women, the Pap test is a regular ritual—slightly unpleasant but necessary for good health. What many don't know is that the Pap test is one of the success stories of modern medicine. The Pap test was named for the physician who invented it, Dr. George N. Papanicolaou of Cornell Medical School. The test started to be vigorously promoted in the United States in the 1940s, and its widespread use has helped to reduce the number of cases of cervical cancer and the death rate from cervical cancer by about 74% between 1955 and 1992.[13,14]

What happens during a Pap test? While a woman lies on an exam table, a physician or nurse inserts a speculum into the patient's vagina to widen it. A sample of cells is taken from the exocervix (the surface of the cervix closest to the vagina) and then from the endocervix (the inside part of the cervix closest to the body of the uterus) with a small spatula, brush, or swab. The specimen, containing cells from the cervix, is placed on a glass slide or rinsed in a vial with a solution that preserves the cells.[14]

The test can detect abnormalities in the cervix that are precancerous, which can be treated, preventing the progression to cervical cancer. It also can detect cervical cancer at a very early stage, when it is most treatable. If abnormal cervical cells are detected early, progression to cervical cancer can be stopped with treatments such as a loop electrosurgical excision procedure (LEEP), in which tissue is removed with a thin wire loop that is heated by electric current and acts as a scalpel.[15] For women whose precancerous cervical lesions are caught early, the 5-year relative survival rate is 100%; for cervical cancers caught at a localized stage, the 5-year relative survival rate is 92%.[11]

This is not to say that the Pap test is perfect. Occasionally, it can miss abnormal cells that may be precancerous or cancerous or may indicate that there are abnormal cells when the cells are actually normal.[16]

Yet the good news is that cervical cancer typically develops over a period of many years. So having Pap tests regularly—repeating the tests every few years according to American Cancer Society guidelines—increases your chances of catching precancers before they turn cancerous or of finding cancer in its early stages. If an abnormality is missed on one test, it generally will be detected with the next Pap test, while the abnormality is still in a precancerous stage.[16]

In the years since the Pap test was first introduced, liquid-based technologies have been introduced. In a traditional Pap test, the cells collected from the cervix are placed on a slide and fixed with a preservative. In a **liquid-based Pap test**, the cells from the cervix are put into a special preservative liquid. Technicians then spread the cells in the liquid onto a glass slide for examination under a microscope. The liquid can help to remove some of the mucus, bacteria, yeast cells, and pus in a sample. It also allows the cervical cells to be spread out more evenly and keeps them from drying out or distorting. Known by brand names such as ThinPrep and AutoCyte, these liquid-based technologies reduce the chances that your Pap test will have to be repeated because of unclear results. Yet the liquid-based tests do not seem to find more precancers than a regular Pap test.[14]

Another new technology developed for the Pap test in recent years is the use of computerized instruments that can spot abnormal cells in cervical samples. Computerized instruments can find abnormal cells that technologists sometimes miss. Many labs now use computerized technology to assess cervical cell samples, although it's not yet known if computerized assessment has a real impact on preventing cervical cancers.[14]

The **human papillomavirus (HPV) DNA test** assesses cervical samples for the DNA of 13 "high risk" types of HPV that can cause cervical cancer. However, it's recommended only for women older than 30 years of age, in combination with the Pap test. It doesn't replace the Pap test as a means of screening for cervical cancer. As noted in Chapter 7, sexually active women in their 20s are much more likely than older women to have an HPV infection that will go away on its own, and the results of the HPV DNA test may not be as significant and may be more confusing for younger women than for older women. The HPV DNA test is also used in women of any age who have slightly abnormal Pap test results to find out if they might need more testing or treatment.

If the test does find that you are infected with HPV but you have a normal Pap smear, it indicates only that you have the virus. You may need to be tested again in 6 to 12 months to see if the virus has cleared. If you have an abnormal Pap smear, as well as a positive test result for HPV, other tests such as a biopsy (to look for precancerous or cancerous changes in the cervix) may be needed.[17,18]

How Can You Make Sure That Your Pap Tests Are as Accurate as Possible?

According to the American Cancer Society,[14] following these guidelines can help:

- Try not to schedule an appointment for a time during your menstrual period. The best time is about 5 days after your menstrual period stops.
- Don't use birth control foams, tampons, jellies, or other vaginal creams for 2 or 3 days before the test.
- Don't douche or have sexual intercourse for 2 days prior to the test.[19]

When To Get a Pap Test

The American Cancer Society updated their guidelines for cervical cancer screening in 2002—guidelines very similar to those of the National

Cancer Institute and the US Preventive Services Task Force. These guidelines say[14,41]

- All women should begin screening about 3 years after they
  start having sex and no later than age 21. A regular Pap test
  should be done every year, Or, if the newer liquid-based Pap
  test is used, testing can be done every 2 years.
- Beginning at age 30, women who have three normal Pap tests
  in a row can be tested less often—every 2 to 3 years.
- If you're older than age 30 and opt to have the Pap test plus the
  HPV DNA test, you can be tested less frequently—about every
  3 years.
- Women who have risk factors for cervical cancer should be
  tested yearly. These include women who were exposed to a
  medication called *diethylstilbestrol* before birth or those with
  a weakened immune system from HIV infection, organ transplant, chemotherapy, or chronic steroid use.
- Women who have had their cervix removed in a total hysterectomy (meaning both the upper part of the uterus and the cervix
  were both removed) can choose to stop cervical cancer testing,
  unless the surgery was done as a treatment for cervical cancer or precancer. Women who have had a partial hysterectomy
  without removal of the cervix need to continue cervical cancer
  screening.
- Women aged 70 years or older with three normal Pap tests in a
  row and no abnormal Pap tests in 10 years can choose to stop
  having cervical cancer tests unless they are at increased risk
  for developing cervical cancer because of diethylstilbestrol
  exposure, HIV infection, or a weakened immune system.
  Women with these conditions should continue to have testing
  as long as they are in good health.

Screening for Colon Cancer: Don't Be Modest

I have to admit that I wasn't looking forward to my first test for colon
cancer when I turned 50. But, with a history of colon cancer in my family,
I knew that this test was vital. The day before the test—the one I chose is
called a **flexible sigmoidoscopy**—I followed a diet that was outlined in
instructions from my health plan and took very strong laxatives as well
as an enema. Needless to say, I went to the bathroom a lot!

The next day, when it was time for the exam, a clinician inserted a sigmoidoscope—a flexible, hollow tube about the thickness of a finger into

my rectum. The sigmoidoscope was gently eased through my colon and had a tiny video camera, which sent pictures to a TV screen. To my surprise, I could see my colon on the TV screen above my head, even as I was undergoing the test. The clinician pointed out that my colon was entirely healthy, without any abnormal growths. "It looks nice and pink," she said.

After the test, which took about 20 minutes, I discarded my hospital dressing gown for my street clothes. I felt reassured that I had been successfully screened for the cancer that had killed my paternal aunt. There are several different tests that are recommended to screen for colorectal cancer, including flexible sigmoidoscopy, and the American Cancer Society recommends that most adults aged 50 years and older should undergo at least one of these tests.[20–22]

The screening tests can be divided into two broad groups:

- *Tests that can find both colorectal polyps and cancer.* These tests look at the structure of the colon to find abnormal areas. This is done either with a scope inserted into the rectum or with special imaging (X-ray) tests. Polyps (benign growths) found before they become cancerous can be removed. Precancerous polyps are known as *adenomas*, and their removal can prevent cancer. The tests that screen for polyps and cancer can prevent colorectal cancer, as well as helping to screen for early cases of cancer. Because of their ability to prevent colorectal cancer, these tests are preferred, if they're available and you're willing to have them. Unless something abnormal is found, they should be repeated every 5 years (for flexible sigmoidoscopy, virtual colonoscopy, and double-contrast barium enema) or every 10 years (for colonoscopy).
- *Tests that mainly find cancer.* These involve testing the stool (feces) for signs that cancer may be present. These tests are less invasive and easier to have done, but they aren't as good as detecting polyps. They also have to be repeated yearly in order to be effective at catching cancer.

Unfortunately, false information and a misplaced sense of modesty have scared people away from these tests. Many people mistakenly believe that tests such as colonoscopy and flexible sigmolidoscopy are painful. In truth, sigmoidoscopy can be somewhat uncomfortable but not painful. During a colonoscopy, you'll usually be given a sedating medication to make sure that you don't experience pain during the test. Some people don't get these tests because they don't want to deal with any test having to do with the rectum. But the fact is that these tests are real lifesavers.

Let's Look at Each of These Tests

Tests that find both colorectal polyps and cancer include[20,22]:

Colonoscopy. A colonoscopy is an exam that allows a doctor to see and look closely at the inside of the entire colon. The colon and rectum are the two parts of the large bowel or large intestine, a muscular tube about 5 feet long involved in storing and removing solid waste (your stool) from the body.

In a colonoscopy, a doctor uses a slender, flexible, hollow, lighted tube to look for cancer or polyps. Polyps are small growths that, over time, can become cancerous. In a colonoscopy, small puffs of air are put into the colon to keep it open and allow the physician to clearly see the colon. Patients are usually given an intravenously administered medicine to help them relax.

Before the test, it's important that the colon and rectum be empty so that your doctor can see them during the test. You may be asked to clean your bowel the night before with laxatives and to stay on a liquid diet for a day before the exam. It's recommend that this test should be done every 10 years.

Virtual Colonscopy. For those who can't have or don't want to have a colonoscopy, there is also a test called a *virtual colonoscopy.* In this test, a computed tomographic (CT) scanner takes pictures as it rotates around you while you lie on a table. A computer then combines these images into "slices" of the part of your body being studied. In a virtual colonoscopy, both two-dimensional X-ray pictures and three-dimensional images of the colon and rectum allow a doctor to check the rectum and colon for polyps or cancer.

The advantages of this test are that it can be done quickly and doesn't require sedation. However, it still requires the same bowel preparation, as well as insertion of a tube into your rectum. And if the clinician sees polyps or other problems on the test, a colonoscopy will be needed to explore the colon more fully or to remove any growths or cancer. It's recommended that this test be performed every 5 years.

Flexible Sigmoidoscopy. A sigmoidoscopy, by contrast, is an exam of only the lower parts of the colon, called the *sigmoid colon* and the *descending colon.* These parts of the colon are examined for signs of cancer or polyps. This exam usually takes about 15 to 20 minutes and can be performed without sedation. Again, small puffs of air are put into the colon to keep it open, which may be only slightly uncomfortable. You'll need to have a bowel preparation to clean out your colon before the test and possibly follow a liquid diet the day before the exam. It's recommended that this test be performed every 5 years.

Double-Contrast Barium Enema. In this test, barium sulfate (a chalky liquid) is used to outline the inner part of the colon and rectum and look for abnormal areas on X-rays. During the test, a flexible tube is inserted into your rectum, and barium sulfate is pumped in to partially fill and open up the colon as you lie on an X-ray table. You'll then be turned on the X-ray table so that the barium spreads throughout the colon. Air is pumped into the colon to make it expand, and X-rays of the lining of the colon are taken. Before the test, you'll need to clean the colon with enemas or laxatives, and you may need to stay on a liquid diet for a day or two beforehand. It's recommended that this test be performed every 5 years.

Tests that mainly find colorectal cancer include[20,22]:

Fecal Occult Blood Test (FOBT).—The FOBT looks for hidden blood in the feces. The idea behind the test is that blood vessels at the surface of larger colorectal polyps or cancers are often fragile and easily damaged by the passage of feces. These damaged vessels usually release a small amount of blood in the feces. The FOBT detects blood in the stool though a chemical reaction. If the test is positive, a colonoscopy is needed to see if there is a cancer or polyps in the colon.

For the FOBT, you use a take-home test in the privacy of your own home. You'll receive a kit that will explain how to take a stool or feces sample, which is usually smeared on small squares of paper, at home. You then mail the kit or take it to a lab for testing. To be most effective, the FOBT should be repeated every year. The FOBT should not be taken during your menstrual period. Before taking an FOBT, your physician may advise you to avoid taking certain medications or eating foods that can affect the test results.

Fecal Immunochemical Test (FIT). Another newer type of test that can detect blood in the stool is FIT. This test is done the same way as an FOBT, but some people find it easier to use because there are no drug or dietary restrictions. The FIT is also done with a take-home kit that provides detailed instructions on how to collect a specimen, with the results evaluated by laboratory staff. Like the FOBT, it should be done every year to be effective. If there's a positive test result, you should undergo a colonoscopy.

Stool DNA Test. Instead of looking for blood in the stool, this test looks for abnormal sections of DNA from cancer or polyps. Cells from colorectal cancer or polyps with these mutations are often shed in the stool, where tests may be able to detect them. Like other stool tests, you'll receive a kit with detailed instructions on how to collect a specimen. It requires you to place an entire stool sample in a special container with an ice pack and pack these into a special shipping box that is sent to the lab for analysis. This is a newer type of test, so it's not clear how often it should be performed. It's also more expensive than other types of stool tests, and like the other stool tests, a colonoscopy will be needed if test results are abnormal.

What if you're at increased risk for colorectal cancer? You should begin screening earlier than age 50 and have the tests more often. These conditions place you at higher than average risk[20]:

- A personal history of colorectal cancer or polyps
- A personal history of inflammatory bowel diseases called *ulcerative colitis* or *Crohn disease*
- A strong family history of colorectal cancer or polyps (Usually this means a diagnosis of colorectal cancer or polyps in any first-degree relative—a parent, sibling, or child. A strong family history also can be indicated by colorectal cancer in two or more first- or second-degree family relatives at any age.)
- A known family history of one of the hereditary or genetic colorectal cancer syndromes, including familial adenomatous polyposis or hereditary nonpolyposis colon cancer (Diagnosis of these syndromes can be based on genetic testing or on personal or family health history.)

If you have any of these conditions, it's important to talk with your healthcare provider about how often you should have screening tests. You may need to have screening tests, such as colonoscopy, as often as every 1 to 2 years, especially if you are genetically at risk for colon cancer. The amount of time between screenings will depend on how high your risk is.[20]

Yet, whether you're at average or increased risk for colorectal cancer, it's important to remember that screening for this disease saves lives. Colorectal cancer is the third leading cause of cancer-related deaths in the United States. And screening is a powerful weapon in preventing colon cancer. The reason is that most colorectal cancers start as polyps, and screening often can find these polyps and allow them to be removed, before they have a chance to turn into cancer. Again, screening also can find colorectal cancer early, when it is most likely to be curable.

One reason why the death rate from colon cancer has been dropping is that more people are getting screened.[21] Treatment for colon cancer also has improved over the years, so there are now more than 1 million colon cancer survivors living in the United States.[23]

Signs and Symptoms of Colorectal Cancer

If you notice any of the following symptoms, you should report them to your doctor right away. They can be signs of colon cancer.

- A change in bowel habits, such as diarrhea, constipation, or a narrowing of the stool that lasts for more than a few days
- A feeling that you need to have a bowel movement, which is not relieved by doing so
- Bleeding from the rectum, dark stools, or blood in the stool
- Cramping or abdominal (stomach) pain
- Weakness and fatigue[22]

Most of these symptoms are usually caused by other conditions that are not cancer, such as hemorrhoids or infection. Still, if you notice any of these problems, it's important to call your doctor right way so that the cause can be found and treated.

Lung Cancer Screening: Why Not?

Whether or not to screen for lung cancer has long been a controversial question. In fact, the effectiveness of screening for lung cancer has been the subject of research for the past 30 years or more.[24,25]

Thirty years ago, several studies found that screening for lung cancer—using a chest X-ray or a sputum sample (in which a sample of mucus brought up from the lungs by coughing is viewed under a microscope to look for cancer cells)—did not improve survival, even when the cancer was found in early stages.[24]

In the 1980s, the American Cancer Society came out with some controversial recommendations. The American Cancer Society advised that doctors no longer do routine chest X-rays as part of the annual physical exam, even for smokers or former smokers.[24] Now, with the availability of spiral CT scans, which allow clinicians to quickly get detailed pictures of the lungs, the controversy over screening for lung cancer has become even more heated. One study by a team of radiologists at Weill Medical

College at Cornell University found that CT scans could indeed find early lung cancers and improve survival rates in smokers and former smokers.[26] However, this study was designed to assess the time period between diagnosis and death (survival) but not whether people who were screened actually lived longer (to an older age) than those who were not.

There are quite a few tests that can find cancer before a patient would have developed symptoms, but only some of these tests find the cancer early enough for cure—to save the patient's life. When tests find cancer early, but not early enough for cure, the result is that the patient learns the bad news sooner. Yet he or she may not really live any longer. And some screening tests lead to a sequence of diagnostic tests and to treatments with serious and even fatal side effects. For these (and other) reasons, knowing that screening improves survival is encouraging—but not enough to recommend a test without further scientific evidence.

The results of some studies on lung cancer screening also came into question when the *New York Times* revealed that the research had been partially underwritten by tobacco companies and that the researchers had 10 pending patents related to CT screening and follow-up technology.[27]

The American Cancer Society and respected organizations such as the American College of Chest Physicians don't recommend widespread lung cancer screening, even for smokers or former smokers.[28,29] The reason is that there is no strong scientific evidence that these screenings actually *save lives*.[28] A large clinical trial known as the National Lung Screening Trial (NLST) is now testing this hypothesis. The trial, which began in 2002, has studied over 50,000 people, and results are expected to be released soon. It's expected that this trial will help to inform us about whether CT scanning can catch lung cancer early enough to save lives.

However, until we know the results of this trial, those at risk for lung cancer should understand the limits and benefits of screening. Studies that also have been updated recently have concluded that X-rays and sputum cytology do not find lung cancers early enough to improve a person's chances for cure. While CT scanning can find lung cancers early, it also can find a lot of abnormalities that turn out not to be cancer. And these findings often lead to a lot of unnecessary testing, biopsies, and even surgery.[28]

Biopsies and operations on the lungs to check for abnormalities found on CT scan or X-ray carry some risk. These biopsies and operations can be fairly invasive and extensive and carry some risk for complications and even for death. A lot of anxiety also can be created when an abnormality is found in the lungs through a CT scan or X-ray, and that anxiety may be unnecessary in patients in whom no cancer is found after biopsy or surgery.

The final choice of whether or not to undergo an annual CT scan is up to individuals and their clinician, and waiting for the results of the National Lung Screening Trial may help to inform this decision. If you are a smoker or former smoker, discuss the benefits and risks of annual CT scans and X-rays with your healthcare provider. Because the benefits of lung cancer screening aren't entirely clear and there are some downsides, you'll have to decide if the chance of finding a lung cancer earlier is worth the drawbacks of undergoing possibly unnecessary tests or operations. Some people would much rather find a lung cancer at an early stage, but others would prefer to avoid unnecessary operations if the benefits of screening aren't proven. Hopefully, the National Lung Screening Trial will provide some answers that can tell us if yearly CT scans for smokers or former smokers would be a wise choice.[28]

Should You Be Screened for Ovarian Cancer?

Ovarian cancer can be a deadly cancer, especially if it's diagnosed after it has spread beyond the ovaries. This cancer is the ninth most common cancer in women[30] and the fourth most common cause of cancer death.[31] When ovarian cancer is caught in its early stages, the 5-year survival rate is good—93%. After the cancer has spread to distant sites, however, the 5-year survival rate drops to 31%.[31] Unfortunately, ovarian cancer is often diagnosed when the cancer is advanced.[32]

What can be done to catch ovarian cancer early? Unfortunately, the screening tests we have for detecting ovarian cancer are imperfect at best. They generate a high rate of false-positive results—meaning that they often falsely indicate cancer that is not there. When a test has a high rate of false-positive results, women who get a "positive" test result may be subjected to invasive procedures to check for cancer—procedures that carry some risk.[32,33] So there would be more harm than benefit in using these tests for screening many women with an average risk of ovarian cancer. In studies of women at average risk for ovarian cancer, screening tests for the disease did not lower the number of deaths either.[34] This is why screening tests for ovarian cancer generally are recommended only for women at high risk of developing the cancer. (These tests are also used for those who have symptoms that suggest they have the disease. When symptoms are present, these tests are not considered screening tests.) Women at high risk include those with a strong family history and those with a *BRCA* mutation that infers increased risk of breast, ovarian, and other cancers. However, even in these women, these tests are problematic, and their use is limited, according to the American Cancer Society.[32] Tests for ovarian cancer include the following:

Transvaginal Ultrasound. In this test, a small instrument is placed inside the vagina, and sound waves emitting from the instrument are used to view the vagina, cervix, uterus, fallopian tubes, and ovaries. The use of transvaginal ultrasound can help your doctor to tell if there is a mass in the ovary, but it can't tell if the mass is cancerous.[34]

Cancer Antigen 125 (CA-125). This blood test looks for levels of a protein that are usually elevated in women with ovarian cancer. The problem with this test is that some conditions other than ovarian cancer also can cause high levels of CA-125. Also, some women with ovarian cancer will have normal CA-125 levels on testing. When a CA-125 test is abnormal, the test often will be repeated to make sure that the result is accurate. If the test is positive, then a transvaginal ultrasound may be ordered or samples of fluid from the abdomen or actual tissue from the ovaries will be taken and tested for cancer.

Proteomic Tests. There has been some promising research toward developing proteomic blood tests for ovarian cancer. These tests (such as OvaSure and OvaCheck) measure many proteins that may be present in higher or lower amounts in women with ovarian cancer. Although some scientists think that this approach may be successful eventually, no proteomic tests for ovarian cancer screening are currently available (except for participants in research studies), none have been proven to be accurate enough to save lives, and none are recommended by the American Cancer Society, other health organizations, or ovarian cancer advocacy groups.[35]

So our best hope for detecting ovarian cancer early is research that improves current screening tests or leads to new methods of early detection that can find ovarian cancer early and save lives.[32] Hopefully, an effective screening test for ovarian cancer, even for women at average risk, will someday be available.

Until that test becomes available, the best way to detect ovarian cancer is to be aware of its symptoms. Unfortunately, the symptoms of ovarian cancer can be similar to those of benign conditions that are more common. However, if you have any of the following symptoms, especially if they are new or persistent, tell your doctor. They may be signs of ovarian cancer.[32]

- Bloating
- Pelvic or abdominal pain

- Difficulty eating or feeling full quickly
- Urinary symptoms, including urgency or frequency, that don't resolve with treatment

If you that think you may have symptoms of ovarian cancer, ask your doctor about testing for the disease.

Prostate Cancer Screening: What You Should Consider

Although there are two methods that can find prostate cancer early—the **prostate-specific antigen (PSA)** blood test and the **digital rectal exam (DRE)**—neither of these methods is perfect. Abnormal results don't always mean that cancer is present, and normal results don't always mean that there is no cancer. Uncertain or false test results can cause confusion and anxiety. Some men also might have a **prostate biopsy,** which has some small risks as well as being uncomfortable, as a result of false-positive DRE or PSA results—when the test falsely indicates that there is cancer. Others might get a false sense of security from normal test or exam results when cancer is actually present.[36]

The PSA test is especially controversial. The PSA test can help to spot many prostate cancers early, but at issue is how dangerous the cancer actually is. Some prostate cancers grow so slowly they would never cause any symptoms or lead to death. But they still might be treated with surgery or radiation because doctors cannot always tell how aggressive the cancer might be. Getting a positive result but no treatment can result in anxiety for the diagnosed men. In addition, treatments for prostate cancer can have side effects, including urinary incontinence and impotence, that can seriously affect a man's quality of life.[36,37]

Since 1992, five years after the PSA was first introduced, prostate cancer death rates have fallen by about 4% per year. However, it's not clear whether this has been due to increased screening rates, improvements in treatment, or both. To date, there have been no studies that have proven that routine screening prevents deaths from prostate cancer.[37,38]

The results of early data from two recent large-scale clinical trials—one American, and one European—have not shed much light on the controversy. The trials, published in the *New England Journal of Medicine* in March, 2009, were designed to test whether prostate cancer screening, including PSA and DRE, would save lives. In the US study of more than 76,000 men, the researchers found no significant difference in prostate cancer death rates between those who did or did not have prostate cancer screening. The European study of 182,000 men found that screening (PSA every 4 years and DRE twice during that same period) reduced the rate of prostate cancer death by 20% after 9 years of follow-up. Yet, according to the scientists who conducted the trial, "1410 men would need to be screened and 48 additional cases of prostate cancer would need to be treated to prevent one death from prostate cancer."[37,39,40]

Thus a small number of men may benefit from prostate screening, but a large number of men also will be treated unnecessarily because of such screening. Because there is no evidence yet that shows conclusively that the benefits of prostate cancer screening outweighs the risks, the American Cancer Society does not recommend routine testing at this time. Along with other cancer organizations, the American Cancer Society recommends that a man's decision of whether or not to undergo prostate cancer screening should be based on a careful conversation with his physician. This conversation should consider the risks and benefits of screening, as well each man's individual medical situation, including his risk for prostate cancer and his values regarding possible side effects.[36,37]

Prostate cancer screening should be discussed with men at average risk starting at age 50. For those at high risk of developing prostate cancer, the discussion about the risks and benefits of screening should take place starting at age 45. Men at high risk include those who are African American and those who have a first-degree relative diagnosed with prostate cancer at an early age (younger than age 65). For men at even higher risk (those with several first-degree relatives with prostate cancer), this discussion should take place at age 40.[36]

Following are descriptions of the PSA and DRE tests and what information they can give you.[36]

PSA Test

The PSA test looks for a substance made by cells in the prostate that is found in both semen and blood. When prostate cancer develops, the PSA level usually goes above 4 ng/mL of blood. However, a lower level sometimes can indicate prostate cancer. About 15% of men with PSA levels below 4 ng/mL will have prostate cancer on biopsy. If you have a PSA level between 4 and 10 ng/mL, however, you have a one in four chance of having prostate cancer. If it's more than 10 ng/mL, your risk of cancer is over 50%.

There are actually a number of factors that can be used to predict prostate cancer risk. Researchers from the University of Texas Health Science Center at San Antonio recently developed an online tool (http://

deb.uthscsa.edu/URORiskCalc/Pages/uroriskcalc.jsp) that estimates prostate cancer risk based on PSA level, family history of prostate cancer, history of prior negative prostate biopsy, DRE results, and race.

"The PSA is not a perfect tumor marker. However, it will pick up cancers well before a physical exam (DRE)," says Joel Nelson, MD, Frederic. N. Schwentker Professor and chairman of the Department of Urology at the University of Pittsburgh Medical Center. Although the classic recommendation is that PSA levels over 4 ng/mL should be investigated, what's often more telling in a PSA test is the increase in value over time. That is, if your PSA level increases significantly from year to year, your doctor may need to do a biopsy. However, even levels below 4 ng/mL may be of concern in younger men and in obese men, who tend to have lower levels of PSA, according to Nelson. At the same time, your PSA level can rise with a number of other conditions than prostate cancer. These include

- *Benign prostatic hyperplasia*, a noncancerous enlargement of the prostate that often occurs as men grow older
- *Prostatitis*, an inflammation or infection of the prostate gland
- *Aging* (PSA levels normally go up as you age.)
- *Ejaculation* (Ejaculation can cause the PSA to go up for a short time and then go down again. This is why some clinicians suggest that men abstain from ejaculation for 2 days before testing.)

Some things also cause PSA levels to go down (even when cancer is present). These include

- *Certain medicines*, such as finasteride or dutasteride, that are used to treat benign prostatic hyperplasia or urinary symptoms
- *Herbal mixtures* (Herbal mixtures sold for "prostate health" also may affect PSA levels and may indicate a normal measurement when your level is actually high. This is why it's important to tell your doctor if you are taking one of these supplements. Saw palmetto does not seem to interfere with PSA measurements.)
- *Obesity* (Obese men tend to have lower PSA levels.)

DRE

Although a DRE is less effective than the PSA test in finding prostate cancer, it can sometimes find cancers in men with normal PSA levels.

This is why the American Cancer Society recommends that when prostate cancer screening is done, both PSA testing and a DRE should be performed.

During the DRE, the doctor inserts a gloved, lubricated finger into the rectum to feel for any bumps or hard areas on the prostate that may be cancer. During this exam, the clinician can feel the prostate gland, which is located in front of the rectum. Since most cancers begin at the back of the gland, cancer sometimes may be spotted during a DRE. Although the exam can be uncomfortable, it doesn't cause pain and takes a short time. The DRE also can be used once a man is known to have prostate cancer to try to see if the disease has spread to nearby tissues or to detect cancer that has come back after treatment.

What Are the Signs of Prostate Cancer?

Prostate cancer is usually found during a PSA test or DRE. The reason is that early prostate cancer usually causes no symptoms. Some advanced cancers can slow or weaken your urinary stream or make you urinate more often, but so can other benign conditions of the prostate. Still, if you have these symptoms, you should report them to your doctor. You also should talk to your doctor right away if you have any of the signs of advanced prostate cancer, including[36]

- Blood in your urine
- Trouble getting an erection
- Pain in the hips, spine, or ribs
- Weakness or numbness in the feet
- Loss of bladder or bowel control

Other diseases also can cause these symptoms, but it's crucial to talk with your doctor if you notice these symptoms.

Screening Tests You Should Consider Having

Table 1 lists common screening tests that you should consider having. Talk with your clinician about these tests, and also talk about if and when you should get them.

Table 1 **American Cancer Society Screening Guidelines for the Early Detection of Cancer in Average-Risk Asymptomatic People**

Cancer Site	Population	Test or Procedure	Frequency
Breast	Women, age 20+	Breast self-examination	Beginning in their early 20s, women should be told about the benefits and limitations of breast self-examination (BSE). The importance of prompt reporting of any new breast symptoms to a health professional should be emphasized. Women who choose to do BSE should receive instruction and have their technique reviewed on the occasion of a periodic health examination. It is acceptable for women to choose not to do BSE or to do BSE irregularly.
		Clinical breast examination	For women in their twenties and thirties, it is recommended that clinical breast examination (CBE) be part of a periodic health examination, preferably at least every 3 years. Asymptomatic women aged 40 and over should continue to receive a clinical breast examination as part of a periodic health examination, preferably annually.
		Mammography	Begin annual mammography at age 40.[*][†]
Colorectal[‡]	Men and women, age 50+	Fecal occult blood test (FOBT)[‡] with at least 50% test sensitivity for cancer, or fecal immunochemical test (FIT) with at least 50% test sensitivity for cancer, or	Annual, starting at age 50

(Continued)

Table 1 American Cancer Society Screening Guidelines for the Early Detection of Cancer in Average-Risk Asymptomatic People (*Continued*)

Cancer Site	Population	Test or Procedure	Frequency
Colorectal[‡]		Stool DNA test	Interval uncertain, starting at age 50
		Flexible sigmoidoscopy, or	Every five years, starting at age 50
		Fecal occult blood test (FOBT)[§] and flexible sigmoidoscopy,[¶] or	Annual FOBT (or or fecal immunochemical test (FIT)) and flexible sigmoidoscopy every five years, starting at age 50
		Double-contrast barium enema (DCBE), or	Every five years, starting at age 50
		Colonoscopy	Every 10 years, starting at age 50
		CT colonography	Every five years, starting at age 50
Prostate	Men, age 50+	Digital rectal examination (DRE) and prostate-specific antigen test (PSA)	Health care providers should discuss the potential benefits and limitations of prostate cancer early detection testing with men and offer the PSA blood test and the digital rectal examina¬tion annually, beginning at age 50, to men who are at average risk of prostate cancer, and who have a life expectancy of at least 10 years.[**]
Cervix	Women, age 18+	Pap test	Cervical cancer screening should begin approximately three years after a woman begins having vaginal intercourse, but no later than 21 years of age. Screening should be done every year with conventional Pap tests or every two years using liquid-based Pap tests. At or after age 30, women who have had three normal test results in

		a row may get screened every two to three years with cervical cytology (either conventional or liquid-based Pap test) alone, or every three years with an HPV DNA test plus cervical cytology. Women 70 years of age and older who have had three or more normal Pap tests and no abnormal Pap tests in the past 10 years and women who have had a total hysterectomy may choose to stop cervical cancer screening.
Endometrial	Women, at menopause	At the time of menopause, women at average risk should be informed about risks and symptoms of endometrial cancer and strongly encouraged to report any unexpected bleeding or spotting to their physicians.
Cancer-related checkup	Men and women, age 20+	On the occasion of a periodic health examination, the cancer-related checkup should include examination for cancers of the thyroid, testicles, ovaries, lymph nodes, oral cavity, and skin, as well as health counseling about tobacco, sun exposure, diet and nutrition, risk factors, sexual practices, and environmental and occupational exposures.

* Beginning at age 40, annual clinical breast examination should be performed prior to mammography.

† ACS recommends annual mammography starting at age 40, whereas some other organizations recommend starting later and/or less frequent testing. (See page 129 for more information).

‡ Individuals with a personal or family history of colorectal cancer or adenomas, inflammatory bowel disease, or high-risk genetic syndromes should continue to follow the most recent recommendations for individuals at increased or high risk.

§ FOBT as it is sometimes done in physicians' offices, with the single stool sample collected on a fingertip during a digital rectal examination, is not an adequate substitute for the recommended at-home procedure of collecting two samples from three consecutive specimens. Toilet bowl FOBT tests also are not recommended. In comparison with guaiac-based tests for the detection of occult blood, immunochemical tests are more patient-friendly, and are likely to be equal or better in sensitivity and specificity. There is no justification for repeating FOBT in response to an initial positive finding.

¶ Flexible sigmoidoscopy, together with FOBT, is preferred, compared to FOBT or flexible sigmoidoscopy alone.

** Information should be provided to men about the benefits and limitations of testing so that an informed decision about testing can be made with the clinician's assistance.

American Cancer Society (ACS) screening guidelines are updated periodically, so please check the ACS Web site for the latest information. An update to the ACS Prostate Cancer Early Detection Guideline was underway as this book was being written.

References

1. American Cancer Society. *Detailed Guide: Breast Cancer—Can Breast Cancer Be Found Early.* Available at www.cancer.org/docroot/CRI/content/CRI_2_4_3X_Can_breast_cancer_be_found_early_5.asp?rnav=cri. Accessed July 17, 2009.

2. American Cancer Society. *Breast Cancer Facts and Figures 2007–2008.* Available at www.cancer.org/docroot/STT/content/STT_1x_Breast_Cancer_Facts_Figures_2007–2008_09.asp. Accessed July 31, 2009.

3. Qaseem A, Snow V, Sherif K, et al. Screening mammography for women 40 to 49 years of age: a clinical practice guideline from the American College of Physicians. *Ann Intern Med.* 2007;146:511–515.

4. Agency for Healthcare Research and Quality, US Preventive Services Task Force. *Screening for Breast Cancer,* November 2009. Available at www.ahrq.gov/clinic/USpstf/uspsbrca.htm#related. Accessed December 1, 2009.

5. Saslow D, Boetes C, Burke W, et al. American Cancer Society guidelines for breast screening with MRI as an adjunct to mammography. *CA Cancer J Clin.* 2007;57:75–89.

6. American Cancer Society. *Breast Cancer: Early Detection.* Available at www.cancer.org/docroot/CRI/content/CRI_2_6x_Breast_Cancer_Early_Detection.asp. Accessed July 31, 2009.

7. American Cancer Society. *Digital Mammograms Outperform Standard Ones in Some Women.* Available at www.cancer.org/docroot/NWS/content/NWS_1_1x_Digital_Mammograms_Outperform_Standard_Ones_in_Some_Women.asp. Accessed July 17, 2009.

8. National Cancer Institute. *Improving Methods for Breast Cancer Detection and Diagnosis.* Available at www.cancer.gov/cancertopics/factsheet/Detection/breast-cancer. Accessed July 17, 2009.

9. National Cancer Institute. *Digital versus Film Mammography in the Digital Mammographic Imaging Screening Trial (DMIST): Questions and Answers.* Available at www.cancer.gov/newscenter/DMISTQandA. Accessed July 17, 2009.

10. American Cancer Society. *Detailed Guide—Breast Cancer. How is Breast Cancer Diagnosed?* Available at www.cancer.org/docroot/CRI/content/CRI_2_4_3X_How_is_breast_cancer_diagnosed_5.asp?rnav=cri. Accessed July 17, 2009.

11. American Cancer Society. *Detailed Guide—Cervical Cancer. What Are the Key Statistics About Cervical Cancer?* Available at www.cancer.org/docroot/CRI/content/CRI_2_4_1X_What_are_the_key_statistics_for_cervical_cancer_8.asp?sitearea=. Accessed July 18, 2009.

12. National Cancer Institute. *Women's Health Report. Cervical Cancer,* March 2003. Available at http://women.cancer.gov/planning/whr0001/cervical.shtml. Accessed July 18, 2009.

13. American Medical Association. *American Medical News. Dr. Pap's Smear: The Test and Its Times,* September 3, 2007. Available at www.ama-assn.org/amednews/2007/09/03/hlsa0903.htm. Accessed July 18, 2009.

14. American Cancer Society. *Cervical Cancer: Prevention and Early Detection.* Available at www.cancer.org/docroot/CRI/content/CRI_2_6X_Cervical_Cancer_Prevention_and_Early_Detection_8.asp?sitearea=&level=. Accessed July 18, 2009.

15. American Cancer Society. *Detailed Guide—Cervical Cancer. Can Cervical Cancer Be Prevented?* Available at www.cancer.org/docroot/CRI/content/CRI_2_4_2X_Can_cervical_cancer_be_prevented_8.asp?rnav=cri. Accessed July 18, 2009.

16. National Cancer Institute. *Pap Test.* Available at www.cancer.gov/cancertopics/factsheet/Detection/Pap-test. Accessed July 18, 2009.

17. National Cancer Institute. *Human Papillomaviruses and Cancer: Questions and Answers.* Available at www.cancer.gov/cancertopics/factsheet/Risk/HPV. Accessed July 18, 2009.

18. American Cancer Society. *Thinking About Testing for HPV?* Available at www.cancer.org/docroot/CRI/content/CRI_2_6x_Thinking_About_Testing_for_HPV.asp?sitearea=&level=. Accessed July 18, 2009.

19. American Cancer Society. *Cervical Cancer: Prevention and Early Detection.* Available at www.cancer.org/docroot/CRI/content/CRI_2_6X_Cervical_Cancer_Prevention_and_Early_Detection_8.asp?sitearea=&level=. Accessed October 21, 2008.

20. American Cancer Society. *Detailed Guide—Colon and Rectum Cancer. Can Colorectal Polyps and Cancer Be Found Early?* Available at www.cancer.org/docroot/CRI/content/CRI_2_4_3X_Can_colon_and_rectum_cancer_be_found_early.asp. Accessed July 18, 2009.

21. Levin B, Lieberman DA, McFarland B, et al. Screening and surveillance for the early detection of colorectal cancer and adenomatous polyps, 2008: a joint guideline from the American Cancer Society, the US Multi-Society Task Force on Colorectal Cancer, and the American College of Radiology. *CA Cancer J Clin.* 2008;58:130–160.

22. American Cancer Society. *Detailed Guide—Colon and Rectum Cancer.* Available at www.cancer.org/docroot/CRI/CRI_2_3x.asp?dt=10. Accessed July 18, 2009.

23. American Cancer Society. *The Cancer Experience: Colon and Rectum Cancer.* Available at www.cancer.org/docroot/CRI/content/CRI_2_8_What_Is_Colon_and_Rectum_Cancer.asp?sitearea=. Accessed July 19, 2009.

24. Lichtenfeld Len, American Cancer Society. *Dr. Len's Cancer Blog. Screening for Lung Cancer: Why Not?* Available at www.cancer.org/aspx/blog/Comments.aspx?id=36. Accessed July 19, 2009.

25. American Cancer Society. *Lung Cancer Screening PDQ.* Health Professional Version. Available at www.cancer.gov/cancertopics/pdq/screening/lung/healthprofessional. Accessed July 31, 2009.

26. Henschke CI, Yankelevitz DF, Libby DM, et al. Survival of patients with stage I lung cancer detected on CT screening. *N Engl J Med.* 2006;355:1763–1771.

27. Harris G. "Cigarette Company Paid for Lung Cancer Study." *New York Times,* March 26, 2008. Available at www.nytimes.com/2008/03/26/health/research/26lung.html. Accessed October 16, 2008.

28. American Cancer Society. *Detailed Guide—Lung Cancer—Non-Small Cell. Can Non-Small Cell Lung Cancer Be Found Early.* Available at www.cancer.org/docroot/CRI/content/CRI_2_4_3x_Can_Non-Small_Cell_Lung_Cancer_Be_Found_Early.asp?sitearea=. Accessed December 1, 2009.

29. American College of Chest Physicians. "New Lung Cancer Guidelines Oppose General CT Screening," press release, September 2007. Available at www.chestnet.org/about/press/releases/2007/070910_1.php. Accessed July 19, 2009.

30. American Cancer Society. *Cancer Statistics 2009.* Available at www.cancer.org/docroot/PRO/content/PRO_1_1_Cancer_Statistics_2009_Presentation.asp. Accessed July 19, 2009.

31. American Cancer Society. *Cancer Facts and Figures 2009.* Available at www.cancer.org/docroot/STT/content/STT_1x_Cancer_Facts__Figures_2009.asp?from=fast. Accessed July 19, 2009.

32. American Cancer Society. *Ovarian Cancer: Why Screening Isn't Routine.* Available at www.cancer.org/docroot/SPC/content/SPC_1_ovarian_Q_A_Saslow.asp. Accessed July 19, 2009.

33. Ferrini R, American College of Preventive Medicine. *Screening Asymptomatic Women for Ovarian Cancer: American College of Preventive Medicine Practice Policy Statement.* Available at www.acpm.org/ovary.htm. Accessed July 19, 2009.

34. American Cancer Society. *Detailed Guide—Ovarian Cancer.* Available at www.cancer.org/docroot/CRI/CRI_2_3x.asp?dt=33. Accessed July 19, 2009.

35. American Cancer Society. *Detailed Guide—Ovarian Cancer. What's New in Ovarian Cancer Research and Treatment?* Available at http://www.cancer.org/docroot/cri/content/cri_2_4_6x_whats_new_in_ovarian_cancer_research_and_treatment_33.asp. Accessed December 2, 2009.

36. American Cancer Society. *Detailed Guide—Prostate Cancer. Can Prostate Cancer Be Found Early?* Available at www.cancer.org/docroot/CRI/content/CRI_2_4_3X_Can_prostate_cancer_be_found_early_36.asp?sitearea=. Accessed July 20, 2009.

37. Snowden RV, American Cancer Society. "Prostate Cancer Screening: Weigh Risks, Benefits with Your Doctor," ACS News Center, March 18, 2009. Available at www.cancer.org/docroot/NWS/content/NWS_1_1x_Prostate_Cancer_Screening_Weigh_Risks_Benefits_With_Your_Doctor.asp. Accessed July 20, 2009.

38. Barry MJ. Screening for prostate cancer—the controversy that refuses to die. *N Engl J Med.* 2009;360:1351–1354.

39. Andriole GL, Crawfor ED, Grubb RL, et al. Mortality results from a randomized prostate-cancer screening trial. *N Engl J Med*. 2009;360:1310–1319.

40. Schroder FH, Hugosson J, Roobol MJ, et al. Screening and prostate-cancer mortality in a randomized European study. *N Engl J Med*. 2009;360:1320–1328.

41. National Cancer Institute. *Cervical Cancer Screening PDQ*. Health Professional Version. Available at www.cancer.gov/cancertopics/pdq/screening/cervical/healthprofessional. Accessed July 31, 2009.

9

The Environment Around Us:
Get the Scoop on Chemicals,
Pollution, and Everyday Products

Chemicals in the environment—including those in the air we breathe, food we eat, water we drink, and products we use—have long been a subject of concern for both scientists and the general public. Scientists agree that exposures to certain chemicals and pollutants do contribute to cancer risk. For instance, asbestos products used as insulating material in buildings are known to increase the risk for lung cancer, especially in workers with heavy exposure to this material.[1] However, the role of some other pollutants and chemicals in causing cancer—especially when exposure to these pollutants occurs at low levels—is debated in the scientific literature.[2]

According to the American Cancer Society, trace levels of pollutants in foods, drinking water, and the air are much less likely to affect your personal cancer risk than factors such as tobacco use, diet, and physical activity.[3] The American Cancer Society estimates that 4% of all cancer deaths are due to occupational exposure to pollutants and 2% to environmental chemicals (such as air pollution). While this may seem like a small number, it's important to consider that 6% of all cancer deaths in the United States corresponds to almost 34,000 cancer deaths, according to 2006 estimates.[1]

The degree of risk from chemicals and pollutants often depends on the concentration and intensity of exposure. For instance, substantial increases in cancer risk have been shown in settings where workers are exposed to high levels of certain chemicals such as arsenic, asbestos, and radon. Yet exposure to some chemicals at low doses, while posing only a small risk to individuals, still can cause substantial ill health across the whole population—whether that comes in the form of cancer risk or other disorders such as respiratory illnesses.[1]

In many ways it can be difficult for scientists to assess the risk posed by chemicals in the environment, especially when they're present at low levels. Most cancers take many years to develop, which makes it difficult to tease out whether a chemical exposure years before contributed to the cancer. Chemicals are also ever present in our environment, so in most cases it's hard to pinpoint one that may have led to an individual diagnosis of cancer. Randomized clinical trials—in which one group of people who receive a new treatment is compared to a second group that does not—are the "gold standard" of cancer prevention and treatment research. Because it obviously would be unethical to intentionally expose groups of people to possible carcinogens in clinical trials, much of our knowledge about which chemicals contribute to cancer risk have come from studies of cells that grow in laboratory dishes and of laboratory animals. We also have gained knowledge by comparing cancer rates among those who've had heavy exposures to certain chemicals or pollutants—for instance, among farmers who use pesticides—with rates in the general population.[4]

Researchers we spoke to for this book indicated that there are certainly chemicals in our environment that have the capacity to cause cancer. But often they alone do not cause the disease. Instead, cancer may be the result of a combination of lifestyle choices, genetic predisposition, and compounds in the environment—all adding up to the damage in our cells that eventually causes cancer. For instance, scientists think that there is a link between tobacco smoking, asbestos exposure, and lung cancer. So workers exposed to asbestos who also smoke have a greater risk of developing lung cancer than they would from either asbestos exposure or smoking alone.

"On an individual basis, it's hard to know what causes a cancer. Chemicals may certainly contribute to cancer, but they're probably not the only causative factor," says Ron Melnick, PhD, toxicologist at the National Institute of Environmental Health Sciences, National Institutes of Health.

Other scientists who study the interrelationship of genetics and environmental chemicals have found that some individuals are more susceptible to these chemicals than the average person, according to Rick Paules, PhD, a senior scientist and head of the Environmental Stress and Cancer Group at the National Institute of Environmental Health Sciences. We'll devote this chapter to answering questions about cancer risk and the environment around us. We'll discuss some of the most common chemicals in our environment—and whether they actually pose a hazard.

Asbestos: A Hazardous Material

Asbestos is a naturally occurring substance that has been definitively linked to lung cancer as well as to *mesothelioma*, a rare cancer of the lining of the chest and abdominal cavities. The International Agency for Research on Cancer (part of the World Health Organization) and the US National Toxicology Program both classify asbestos as a known human carcinogen.[5] The most common use of asbestos has been as an insulating material in buildings and ships since ancient times. The connection between asbestos and lung cancer was noted in scientific studies as early as 1925 and has been confirmed by many studies of exposed workers, especially those who worked in shipbuilding and construction industries. Asbestos use is now restricted, but workers employed in construction, electrical work, or carpentry still may be exposed through renovations or asbestos removal projects.[1,5]

People are usually exposed to asbestos when they inhale fibers in the air. Asbestos fibers can create a dust that is composed of tiny particles that float in the air. This dust can occur when asbestos insulation is installed or when older asbestos-containing materials begin to break down. There is very little danger to health as long as the asbestos is contained in an intact product, such as ceiling tiles. Asbestos exposure becomes a concern, however, when the material is damaged or disturbed—for instance, by drilling or remodeling.[1]

Asbestos use has declined since the mid-1960s when alternative insulating materials were developed. However, exposure to asbestos can be problematic during renovation or demolition of older buildings built before 1975. Because of the hazards associated with the presence of asbestos, contractors involved in removal or other uses of asbestos must be specially licensed and comply with federal, state, and local laws. Workers renovating old buildings who may be exposed to asbestos should use special masks and other protective equipment. Because it's a well-recognized human carcinogen, it's important to get a health checkup from a doctor experienced with asbestos-related diseases if you think you have been heavily exposed to asbestos.[5]

It's also important to assess the amount of your exposure. If you were exposed only briefly or only at low levels, your risk of resulting disease is minimal. But those with heavy asbestos exposure should have regular chest X-rays and lung function tests. It's also important to get prompt attention for any respiratory illness. Smokers are much more susceptible than nonsmokers to asbestos-related illnesses, so it is very important for smokers concerned about asbestos exposure to quit.[1]

Radon: An Invisible Carcinogen

Radon is a colorless, odorless radioactive gas present both indoors and outdoors. It forms from the decay of naturally occurring uranium-238, which is found in soil and rock throughout the world. Exposure in homes usually results from radon that rises from the soil. After smoking, radon exposure is the second leading cause of lung cancer in the United States.[6] If you're a smoker and you also have high levels of radon in your home, you are at especially high risk for lung cancer.[7,8] The International Agency for Research on Cancer and the US National Toxicology Program both classify radon as a known human carcinogen.[7]

Exposure to radon is a known cause of lung cancer in underground miners of uranium and other ores. Indoor exposure is usually at far lower levels than the occupational exposure for miners. However, some contaminated homes have been found to have levels of radon that exceed those in mines. The US Environmental Protection Agency (EPA) estimates that as many as one in 15 homes in the United States has elevated radon levels. Radon levels are usually highest in the basement, which is closest to the soil that releases radon-containing gas. When there's little ventilation, radon can build up and reach high levels.[7,8]

The good news is that radon exposure can be assessed readily. You can purchase radon detection kits in hardware or home-supply stores, or you can hire an expert. Do-it-yourself kits are placed in the home and then mailed to a lab for analysis. The EPA recommends that radon levels should not be above 4 pCi/L and ideally should be 2 pCi/L or below. This measurement evaluates the units of radioactivity per volume of air. If radon levels are above what the EPA recommends, you can reduce levels in your home by installing special ventilation and by sealing cracks in the foundation, floors, and walls. A qualified contractor for reducing radon in your home can be found through the EPA Web site at www.epa.gov/iaq/contacts.html. You can find general information about radon in your area by contacting your state radon office. But remember that radon levels in the same area can vary greatly from home to home. Contact information for these offices can be found at www.epa.gov/iaq/whereyoulive.html.[7,8]

Outdoor Air Pollution and Cancer

Outdoor air pollution is a mixture of substances that come from different sources—including cars, buses, and trains as well as industrial sources, such as fossil fuel–powered electrical generating plants and incinerators.[1]

Exposure to air pollution has been associated with a number of health risks, including respiratory problems and heart disease.[1] A 2009 report from the EPA based on emissions data from 2002 found that 80 different pollutants are thought to affect cancer risk. However, the good news is that the lifetime risk of developing cancer from pollution has decreased since the last EPA analysis of emissions was published in 2006. The new report found that one out of every 27,000 Americans would develop cancer because of breathing polluted air—if those individuals were exposed to 2002 emissions levels 24 hours a day for 70 years. In real terms, the EPA report shows that for every million people an additional 36 would be diagnosed with cancer. To put this in context, in the United States, about 406,000 out of every 1 million people will develop cancer during their lifetime. Air pollution would add 36 cases to this number. While this is a small percentage of those who get cancer, air pollution is still a serious concern, especially because it causes other health problems.[9]

The cancer that has been most strongly linked to air pollution is lung cancer. One 2002 study published in the *Journal of the American Medical Association*,[10] based on data from the American Cancer Society's Cancer Prevention II study, found that exposure to fine particles in air pollution increased the risk of both heart disease and lung cancer. The risk comes from a combination of gases from auto exhaust and smokestacks that combines with oxygen in the air to form very small particles that are then breathed in. The 2002 report found that breathing very polluted air long term can raise the risk of lung cancer as much as breathing second-hand smoke.[11]

The new EPA report found that emissions from vehicles were responsible for 30% of the cancer risk owing to air pollution, and local industry emissions accounted for 25% of the air pollution risk. The data in the EPA report will be used to help states shape air quality control plans required by the Clean Air Act, which gives states the responsibility for regulating air pollution. Since the Clean Air Act was passed in 1990, toxic air emissions have decreased by 40%, according to the EPA.[9]

Diesel exhaust, a type of air pollution that is a concern especially for people who may be heavily exposed, such as railroad workers and truck drivers, comes from diesel engines in trucks, buses trains, ships, construction and farm equipment, and some cars. Some studies of workers exposed to diesel exhaust have found small but significant increases in lung cancer. Diesel exhaust also may be linked to cancers of the larynx, pancreas, bladder, and kidney. The International Agency for Research on Cancer and the US National Toxicology Program include diesel exhaust on their lists of probable human carcinogens.[12] If you think that you have been or are being heavily exposed to diesel fumes, there are some protective measures that you can take. These include[12]

- Checking with your employer to make sure that worker protection policies are in place, such as providing adequate ventilation
- Changing clothes after work and washing hands regularly
- Keeping food out of the work area

The Scoop on Arsenic

You may think of arsenic as a poison that is used only in murder plots of Agatha Christie novels and TV shows. But arsenic-containing compounds are found in industry and occur naturally in some water supplies. Arsenic compounds have been used in wood preservatives, insecticides, herbicides, glass manufacturing, and even some medicines (usually for veterinary use). The main occupational exposure nowadays involves production and use of arsenic-treated wood. Community exposure to arsenic can occur near wood-preservative or glass factories. And people who live in areas where arsenic is found naturally at high levels in drinking water may take in dangerous amounts over the course of a lifetime. Water in areas in some parts of the United States, particularly in the rural western United States, contains some arsenic. However, arsenic levels in public drinking water are regulated. The maximum contaminant level for inorganic arsenic permitted in US drinking water is 10 µg/L. Even in areas of the United State where levels in well water are above the EPA's guidelines, studies to date have not found a significant link between arsenic exposure and cancer.[13]

Studies have found that arsenic can cause lung cancer in highly exposed workers and lung, skin, bladder, and kidney cancers in communities with highly contaminated water. However, most areas with high levels of arsenic in the water are located in other countries, such as Taiwan, China, and Argentina.[13] Arsenic is on the International Agency for Research on Cancer and the US National Toxicology Program lists of known human carcinogens.[13]

Very little arsenic escapes from wood products, and these products are not considered dangerous for adults. However, some scientists note that it's safest for children to use playground equipment that hasn't been treated with wood preservatives containing arsenic. Some also recommend that children wash their hands with soap and water after playing on playground equipment made with arsenic-preserved wood and that builders do likewise after working with this material.[13]

Benzene and Cancer Risk

Benzene is a chemical that is used widely in the United States.[14] It's used as a liquid solvent, as a starting material for the synthesis of other chemicals, and as a gasoline additive. The greatest risk of high-level benzene exposure occurs in the workplace—in industries that make or use benzene, such as the rubber industry, oil refineries, chemical plants, shoe manufacturers, and gasoline-related industries.[15]

Sources of benzene in the environment include gasoline, automobile exhaust fumes, cigarette smoke, emissions from industrial processes, and waste water from some industries. While benzene is found in air in urban and rural areas, the levels are usually very low. Benzene is produced when tobacco burns. Between 50 and 150 µg of benzene is released per cigarette, so smoking and secondhand smoke are important sources of exposure. Some household products such as glues, cleaning products, detergents, art supplies, and paint strippers contain benzene.[12,15]

Workers exposed to high levels of benzene have an increased risk of leukemia, primarily acute myeloid leukemia, and to a lesser degree chronic lymphocytic leukemia. The International Agency for Research on Cancer rates benzene as a known human carcinogen.[15]

If you are concerned about benzene exposure, there are three ways to limit your exposure, according to the American Cancer Society[15]:

- If you're exposed on the job or when using products with benzene, try to replace benzene with another solvent or use personal protective equipment.
- If you're a smoker, stop smoking because smoking increases blood levels of benzene.
- Avoid gasoline fumes by pumping gasoline carefully, and choose gas stations with vapor-recovery systems that capture the fumes.

Drycleaning and Cancer

Another chemical that that can affect health and the environment is called *perchloroethylene*, or *perc*, also known as *tetrachloroethylene*. Many drycleaners use perc to clean garments. Clothes at drycleaners are cleaned in a liquid solution that is mostly perc or some other solvent, sometimes along with a small amount of water. However, perc is a toxic chemical and is classified as a probable human carcinogen by both the International Agency for Research on Cancer and the US National Toxicology Program.[16,17]

The link between perc and cancer has been investigated in scientific studies. In laboratory studies, perc causes cancer in rats. There's also some evidence that workers in the laundry and drycleaning industry are subject to elevated risk of certain kinds of cancers, particularly lung, esophageal, and cervical cancer, although these studies did not consider the impact of lifestyle factors (such as smoking and alcohol consumption) in these workers. However, the risk for cancer also depends on how much exposure a person has, how often the exposure occurs, and how long it lasts.[16,17]

It's thought that the low levels of perc found in the air and drinking water nationwide are not a hazard to human health. It is also unlikely for a person to get cancer from having his or her clothes drycleaned. As part of the drycleaning process, the cleaners remove the perc from the drycleaned clothes, so unless you're in the drycleaning business, there's little reason to think that perc from your drycleaning can affect your cancer risk.[17]

Factors that can elevate workers' exposure to perc include poorly maintained machines, equipment leaks, clothes that are not properly dried or processed, and older machines. New drycleaning equipment and good cleaning practices can reduce workers' exposure to perc significantly.[17]

In addition to these human health concerns, leaky pipes or improper disposal can contaminate the groundwater with perc and can harm plants and aquatic animals.

Some drycleaners do not use perc, instead electing to use a sophisticated machine-based process called *wetcleaning*, which uses water as the solvent. Wetcleaning is done using specialized machines and specially formulated detergents and additives to wash and dry clothes. Although wetcleaning seems appealing from an environmental point of view, there are still unanswered questions about the impact of the processes used. Wetcleaning uses more water and energy than drycleaning, and wetcleaning detergents and additives often end up going down the drain.[17]

To find more information about wetcleaning and to get a list of cleaners nationwide that use the process, you can call the Pollution Prevention Information Clearinghouse at 202–566-0799 and ask for the EPA publication, "Wetcleaning."[17]

What Are Endocrine Disruptors, and Do They Cause Cancer?

Endocrine disruptors are chemicals, both natural and manufactured, that may interfere with the endocrine system in humans and animals.[18]

Pesticides: The Debate About Cancer Risk

In recent years, there are few environmental issues that have stirred up as much public controversy as pesticides. Pesticides are chemicals used to eliminate or control unwanted or harmful insects, plants, fungi, animals, or microorganisms. They're often used in agriculture to protect food crops and plants. The International Agency for Research on Cancer has concluded that some substances used in pesticides are known, probable, or possible carcinogens and that occupational use of some insecticides is probably carcinogenic.[19,20]

Scientific studies of people with high exposures to pesticides, such as farmers and pesticide applicators, have found high rates of blood and lymphatic system cancers; cancers of the lip, stomach, lung, brain, and prostate; and melanoma and other skin cancers, according to the National Cancer Institute. Pesticides such as DDT (which is now banned but was used in agriculture in the past) degrade slowly and can lead to accumulation in the food chain and persistent residues in body fat. These residues have been suggested as a possible risk factor for breast cancer, although the majority of the evidence does not support an association.[14,19,21]

Certainly, some people such as farmers, pesticide applicators, crop dusters, pesticide manufacturers, and even home gardeners can be at risk of high exposure to pesticides, according to the National Cancer Institute.[19]

The controversy over pesticides, however, lies in whether or not exposure to low levels of these chemicals is dangerous in terms of cancer risk.[22] Most people are exposed to low levels of pesticides through use of insect repellents and residues on vegetables and fruit bought in the supermarket. According to the American Cancer Society, the low concentrations of pesticides in some foods have not been associated with increased cancer risk. People who eat more fruits and vegetables, which may be contaminated with trace amounts of pesticides, for instance, generally have lower cancer risk than those who eat few of these foods.[21]

A 2004 review by scientists from the National Cancer Institute and the National Institute for Environmental Health considered the health effects of chronic pesticide exposure after assessing a large number of published studies. Although some studies found a link between pesticide use and cancers such as non-Hodgkin lymphoma, leukemia, multiple myeloma, and cancers of the pancreas, lung, and ovaries, the scientists noted that studies on environmental exposure to pesticides and cancer risk often have suffered from inadequate assessments of exposure. So the results of these studies have been called into question. "Only arsenic-containing insecticides (which have been discontinued in the United States) are recognized as carcinogenic in humans, although many others are suspected human carcinogens," they said.[23]

So, while the weight of the evidence does not suggest that residues of pesticides on foods increase an individual's cancer risk, you still can reduce exposure by washing these foods thoroughly. Some people also prefer organic foods—those grown without pesticides—although there is no research that demonstrates whether these foods are more effective in reducing cancer risk than those grown with traditional methods.[24]

These chemicals are found in many of the everyday products we use, including some plastic bottles, metal food cans, detergents, foods, toys, cosmetics, and pesticides. One example is *bisphenol A* (BPA), a chemical used in some plastic products. Although there is limited information about the effects of these chemicals on human health, there is concern about them because—although they're present in the environment at low levels—they've been shown to have adverse effects on wildlife and in laboratory animals even at these low levels.

Some scientists think that these chemicals adversely affect health, resulting in decreased fertility and possibly in cancers, such as those of the breast and prostate. The difficulty in assessing public health effects, however, is that people are simultaneously exposed to multiple endocrine disruptors, as well as many other chemicals. Thus it's difficult to assess exactly how these chemicals affect human health.

It's thought that endocrine disruptors pose the greatest risk during prenatal and early postnatal development (when animals or humans are developing in the womb or as infants). For instance, researchers have found that animals exposed to low doses of BPA during fetal development are more likely to develop types of precancers that can lead to cancer of the prostate and breast. Although there is little evidence yet that low-dose exposure to this chemical or other endocrine disruptors causes cancer in humans, research is continuing on these chemicals.

A Hard Plastic and Some Hard Questions: BPA

Recently, scientists have raised concerns over the possible health effects of BPA.[25] BPA is used widely in consumer plastic products, including some plastic water and baby bottles, the lining of food cans, food packaging, and compact discs. In a report from the US National Toxicology Program, experts noted "some concern" about the effects of BPA on infants and children and called for more research into the question of whether it affects human health.

However, most of the evidence about the harm from BPA has come from animal studies. When pregnant rats were injected with BPA, their female pups showed breast tissue changes that some researchers suspected might eventually progress to breast cancer, and male pups showed prostate tissue changes that researchers thought might lead to prostate cancer. In some studies, the mice also entered puberty earlier than normal; in humans, early puberty is linked to higher breast cancer risk. However, the report from the US National Toxicology Program also noted that it's difficult to apply the results of these experiments to humans and to know what the result of BPA exposure on humans may be. One problem is that the animals in these experiments were not followed long enough to see if cancer developed, and the mice were exposed to BPA (by injection) in different ways than are humans, who are exposed mainly though food.

Most people are exposed to only trace amounts of the chemical. In addition, not all plastic containers have BPA. Those that do are usually hard and unbreakable and should be marked by the recycling number 7 on the bottom or the letters PC (for *polycarbonate*). Until very recently, plastic containing BPA was used for the majority of hard plastic baby bottles and sports water bottles. However, the majority of plastic bottles do not currently contain or leach BPA, according to Michael Shelby, PhD, director of the National Toxicology Program Center for the Evaluation of Risks to Human Reproduction, part of the National Institute of Environmental Health Sciences. Shelby also notes that most plastic containers made to store food do not contain BPA. It is presently thought that most human exposure actually comes through the lining of canned foods.

Should you be wary of BPA? It's probably prudent to limit your exposure until more is known about this chemical. You can do this by limiting canned beverages, fruits, and vegetables when fresh or frozen products are available as substitutes. You can use glass, porcelain, and stainless-steel containers for hot foods and liquids. At high temperatures, BPA is more likely to leach out of plastic. Although most foods that come in microwave containers are safe, you may want to transfer foods packaged with plastic containing BPA to another container before microwaving them. You also can use baby and water bottles that are BPA-free.[26]

Cancer and Cell Phones

Recently, there's been some publicity about a possible link between cell phone use and brain tumors. Cell phones are ubiquitous, and brain cancer is a serious disease, so this is a topic of some concern. Cellular phones became widely used in the 1990s. So, although they have been studied extensively, we don't yet have information on the potential health effects of long-term use or use by children. Some small studies have shown an association between cell phone use and the risk of brain tumors, but the largest and most reliable studies have not shown such a link. Most large studies have not found that patients with brain tumors have used cell phones more than those without brain tumors when the two groups were compared. None of the studies showed a *dose-response relationship* either—a tendency for the risk of brain tumors to increase with increasing cell phone use. Also, most, but not all, of the studies have not found an association between the side of the head on which the brain tumor occurred and the side on which the cell phone was used.[27]

Acoustic neuroma—a rare slow-growing tumor of the acoustic nerve (which transmits sensation of hearing from the ear to the brain)—also has been studied for a possible link to cell phone use. Results of these studies have been inconsistent. One of the largest and most recent studies, which analyzed data from five European countries, however, found no association between cell phone use, duration of use, or number of calls made and acoustic neuroma.[27]

Wireless devices do emit low levels of radiofrequency energy, similar to that emitted by a microwave oven. According to the US Food and Drug Administration (FDA) and Federal Communications Commission (FCC), most studies of exposure to low levels of radiofrequency energy have not found any adverse health effects. However, you also should consider that not all scientific studies about cell phones and cancer agree. According to the FDA and FCC, the risk from cell phones—if any—is likely to be quite small. But, if you'd like to be cautious, you can try using an earpiece, which would keep the phone's antenna away from your head. Or you can try limiting your calls on your cell phone.

The use of cell phones starting at a young age conceivably could be cause for concern. If there are health effects, they might be more pronounced in children because their nervous systems are still developing. And by starting phone use at a younger age, children are also likely to have a much higher total lifetime exposure. So, for parents, cell phone use by children could be limited, or cell phones could be used with an earpiece.[27]

As far as cell phone towers and cancer, there is little evidence of any harm. Theoretically, cell phone towers are unlikely to cause cancer because the energy level of the radio waves emitted by these towers is relatively low, according to the American Cancer Society. Most public exposure near cell phone towers is similar to that from radio and broadcast TV stations. Animal studies generally have not shown a cancer-causing effect from radio waves.[28]

What's the Risk: Answers to Common Questions About the Environment and Cancer

Here's a look at some common questions about environmental carcinogens and what the American Cancer Society, the FDA and US Department of Health and Human Services say about these chemicals and products.

Do Hair Dyes Cause Cancer?

Studies have looked at whether people who use hair-dye products or those who regularly work with them have an increased risk of various kinds of cancer. The evidence from these studies is inconsistent. Although some studies show a link between hair dyes and cancer, others do not.[29]

There are several different types of hair dyes, including temporary, semipermanent, and permanent hair dyes. Permanent hair dyes cause chemical changes in the hair shaft. There are two types of permanent hair dyes: oxidative and progressive hair dyes. Oxidative dyes use colored dyes and hydrogen peroxide, and progressive dyes contain metal salts. Concern about cancer risk is largely limited to semipermanent dyes and oxidative hair dyes, especially dark brown and black dyes.[29]

If you'd like to reduce your exposure to hair dyes, here are some suggestions from the FDA[29]:

- Don't leave the dye on your head any longer than necessary, and rinse your scalp thoroughly after use.
- Use gloves when applying the dye, and follow the directions on the package.
- Never mix hair-dye products, and do a patch test to check for allergic reactions before use.
- Never dye your eyebrows or eyelashes.

- Delay dying your hair until later in life when it starts to turn gray.
- Consider using henna, which is plant-based, or hair dyes that are lead acetate–based.

Is There Danger From Electromagnetic Fields?

Electromagnetic fields are emitted from devices that produce, transmit, or use electrical power. Some sources of electromagnetic fields are power lines and transmitters, computer monitors, televisions, electric blankets, and many other household devices. Extensive studies have evaluated the exposure of children and adults to electromagnetic fields and the risk of brain tumors and leukemia. Studies of electric utility workers have shown a minimal increase in the risk of brain tumors and leukemia. These increases could be a sign of increased cancer risk, or they could be due to chance alone, according to the American Cancer Society. Results from studies of childhood leukemia and electromagnetic fields have been inconsistent. In 1999, the National Institute of Environmental Health Sciences released results of an extensive 6-year study that stated that the evidence of cancer from exposure to power lines is "weak," but efforts to reduce exposure, when possible, should continue.[30]

Do Growth Hormones Used in Cows to Increase Milk Production Lead to Cancer?

Recombinant bovine growth hormone (rBGH) is a synthetic hormone that is marketed to dairy farmers to increase milk production. The use of rBGH was approved by the FDA in 1993, but it has been banned in the European Union and Canada since 1999.[31]

Some studies have shown that adults who drink milk have about 10% higher levels of insulin-like growth factor 1 (IGF-1) in the blood than those who drink little or no milk. Substantial evidence indicates that IGF levels at the high end of the normal range may influence the development of some tumors, such as breast, prostate, and colorectal cancers. However, there is no evidence that drinking milk—produced with or without rBGH treatment—increases blood IGF levels into the range of concern. There have been no studies comparing IGF-1 levels in people who drink ordinary milk versus those who drink milk stimulated by rBGH. And drinking soy milk also seems to increase levels of IGF-1 in the blood, suggesting that this finding is unlikely to be related to cow's milk or rBGH. Thus far, therefore, there is no evidence that drinking milk from cows treated with rBGH has any effect on cancer risk. Although rBGH is approved in the United States, demand for it has decreased in recent years. Fewer than one in five cows is being injected with rBGH, according to a 2007 US Department of Agriculture survey.[31]

Does Water Fluoridation Cause Cancer?

Fluorides are compounds that are found in drinking water. These compounds were added to the water supply beginning in 1945, when scientists noted that people living in areas with higher water fluoride levels had fewer cavities. Fluoride compounds include the element fluorine with another substance, usually a metal. Examples include sodium fluoride, stannous fluoride, and fluoride monofluorophosphate (MFP). Studies have looked at whether fluoride causes cancer in both animals and humans. So far, most studies have not found a strong link between water fluoride levels and cancer. The International Agency for Research on Cancer has noted that the available scientific evidence is inadequate to draw conclusions about whether or not fluoride increases the risk of cancer. Scientific reviews of recent studies also have concluded that the weight of the evidence does not support a link between fluoride exposure and increased cancer risk in humans.[32]

Do Some Medicines Increase Cancer Risk?

Some medicines we take do increase cancer risk. For instance, some chemotherapy drugs used to treat cancer can increase the risk of second cancers later in life. At the same time, taking chemotherapy treatment when recommended by evidence-based clinical guidelines is well worth the tradeoff. Chemotherapy medicines can cure some people with cancer and extend the lives of some others—and for most people, they do this without incurring second cancers.[33]

Drugs that suppress the immune system—used to treat some cancers as well as to prepare patients for receiving organ transplants—also are associated with an increased risk of cancer, particularly lymphoma. However, the lifesaving benefits of these drugs outweigh the risk for cancer years later, according to the FDA.[33]

The truth is that any medication carries risks and benefits, so be sure to check with your healthcare provider about side effects and complications of any new drug.

One type of medicine that has received a lot of attention in recent years has been *postmenopausal hormone therapy,* also known as *hormone-replacement therapy* (HRT)—a medication that is a combination of the hormones progestin and estrogen. Women used HRT for decades because it relieved menopause symptoms, such as hot flashes. Estrogen by itself can relieve symptoms of menopause, but it can increase a woman's risk of endometrial (uterine lining) cancer, as well as ovarian cancer. So, for many years, most women with a uterus took combined HRT after menopause, which provided the benefits of estrogen without the risk of endometrial cancer. Many doctors once thought that these medications protected against heart disease as well. However, recent studies have found that these medicines are associated with an increased risk for heart disease, stroke, and serious blood clots. These studies also have highlighted the issue of cancer risk associated with HRT.[34]

What do the studies say about HRT and a woman's risk of cancer?

- Results from the Women's Health Initiative study (a large study that assessed HRT use in women and its effects) and other studies have shown that daily use of combined HRT modestly increases a woman's chance of breast cancer with each year of use. Doctors think that much of the risk of breast cancer comes from the progestin in HRT. Scientists are now evaluating whether the dose of progestin can be lowered while still protecting from endometrial cancer.
- Whether HRT increases ovarian cancer risk is still uncertain.
- The Women's Health Initiative study found that using combined HRT increased the risk of dying from lung cancer, although the risk of developing lung cancer was not higher. More studies are needed to confirm this risk.
- The Women's Health Initiative study also concluded that combined HRT reduced the risk of colorectal cancer by about 40%. But some other medications, as well as screening tests for precancerous polyps, also can reduce colorectal cancer risk. HRT is not recommended for this purpose.[34]

HRT also can be used to treat osteoporosis as well as menopause symptoms. But so can other, safer medications. Whether or not you use HRT should be a decision made with your doctor after weighing the possible benefits and risks. If you decide to use HRT, it is usually best to use it at the lowest dose possible and for as short a time as possible. You should consider your risk factors for cancer in your decision, as well as your risk factors for osteoporosis, heart disease, and stroke. You also should consider the severity of your menopause symptoms and whether other medications can help. Some women, for instance, can get relief from hot flashes by taking certain antidepressants, such as fluoxetine (Prozac).[34]

Medical Radiation and Cancer Risk

Medical radiation is used for diagnostic X-rays and computed tomographic (CT) scans as well as for radiation therapy. Radiation therapy is used to treat some types of cancers and involves dosages many thousands of times higher than those used in diagnostic X-rays or CT scans.[33]

Most studies on the long-term effects of exposure to radiation from X-rays to diagnose or screen for cancers or other diseases have not shown an elevated cancer risk. One study published in the *New England Journal of Medicine* in 2007, however, raised concerns when it noted that the typical doses of radiation used in diagnostic CT scans might cause a slight increase in cancer risk. This issue may not be as concerning for adults because cancers that result from a CT scan could take many years or even decades to develop. However, it may be more of a concern for children who receive CT scans. Still, the bottom line is that the potential cancer risk from a single CT scan for an individual person is very small, according to the American Cancer Society. And often the potential benefits outweigh the risks. However, it's wise to follow a few precautions when getting a CT scan[35,36]:

- Ask your doctor whether you really need the scan and whether it will make a difference in your treatment.
- Make sure that the scan is done on modern equipment, and ask that the machine be set for the lowest radiation dose for your particular scan and circumstances.
- Ask if there is another test—such as an ultrasound or magnetic resonance imaging (MRI)—that can provide the same information with less radiation risk.[35]

Finally, remember that CTs are a *very useful* tool for diagnosing disease, including cancer, and any risk from them is likely to be very small.[35]

Some studies have associated radiation therapy with an increased risk of thyroid cancer and early-onset breast cancer, although the risk is considered small. The reason is that most radiation is used in a localized or confined area, which means fewer normal cells are exposed to radiation. Usually the benefits of radiation therapy for cancer outweigh the risks.[30,33]

Treatment for Hodgkin disease, a type of lymphoma, however, delivers low radiation doses to many areas of the body. Patients with Hodgkin disease *are* at increased risk for secondary tumors, such as breast cancer. Studies also have found that people treated with radiation therapy in childhood for acne, ringworm, and other head and neck conditions may be at increased risk for thyroid cancer and other tumors of the head and neck (although radiation has not been used as a treatment for these conditions for many years). Be sure to talk with your doctor about how often you should have screening tests for cancer if you've had treatment for Hodgkin disease or radiation therapy for other conditions in childhood.[30,33] (For more information on preventing cancer for cancer survivors, see Chapter 11.)

References

1. American Cancer Society. *Cancer Facts and Figures 2006. Special Section: Environmental Pollutants and Cancer.* Available at www.cancer.org/downloads/STT/CAFF2006PWSecured.pdf. Accessed July 22, 2009.

2. Clapp RW, Howe GK, Jacobs MM. Environmental and occupational causes of cancer: a call to act on what we know. *Biomed Pharmacother.* 2007;61:631–639.

3. American Cancer Society. "The Environment and Cancer Risk." ACS News Center, January 14, 2000. Available at www.cancer.org/docroot/NWS/content/NWS_2_1x_The_Environment_and_Cancer_Risk.asp. Accessed July 22, 2009.

4. Mayo Foundation for Medical Education and Research. *Carcinogens in the Environment: A Major Cause of Cancer?* MayoClinic.com, May 24, 2006. Available at www.riversideonline.com/health_reference/Cancer/CA00076.cfm. Accessed July 22, 2009.

5. American Cancer Society. *Asbestos.* Available at www.cancer.org/docroot/PED/content/PED_1_3X_Asbestos.asp?sitearea=PED. Accessed July 22, 2009.

6. American Cancer Society. "Radon Risk for Lung Cancer Back in the Spotlight." ACS News Center, February 9, 2005. Available at www.cancer.org/docroot/NWS/content/NWS_2_1x_Radon_Risk_for_Lung_Cancer_Back_in_the_Spotlight.asp. Accessed July 22, 2009.

7. American Cancer Society. *Radon.* Available at www.cancer.org/docroot/PED/content/PED_1_3x_Radon.asp?sitearea=PED. Accessed July 22, 2009.

8. US Environmental Protection Agency. *A Citizen's Guide to Radon.* Available at www.epa.gov/radon/pdfs/citizensguide.pdf. Accessed July 22, 2009.

9. Snowden RV, American Cancer Society. "EPA Estimates Cancer Risk Associated with Air Pollution." ACS News Center, June 25, 2009. Available at www.cancer.org/docroot/NWS/content/NWS_1_1x_EPA_Estimates_Cancer_Risk_Associated_With_Air_Pollution.asp. Accessed July 23, 2009.

10. Pope CA, Burnett RT, Thun MJ, et al. Lung cancer, cardiopulmonary mortality, and long-term exposure to fine particulate air pollution. *JAMA.* 2002;287:1132–1141.

11. American Cancer Society. "Air Pollution Linked to Deaths from Lung Cancer." ACS News Center, March 6, 2002. Available at www.cancer.org/docroot/NWS/

content/NWS_1_1x_Air_Pollution_Linked_to_Deaths_From_Lung_Cancer. asp. Accessed July 23, 2009.

12. American Cancer Society. *Diesel Exhaust.* Available at www.cancer. org/docroot/PED/content/PED_1_3x_Diesel_Exhaust.asp?sitearea=PED. Accessed July 23, 2009.

13. American Cancer Society. *Arsenic.* Available at www.cancer.org/docroot/ PED/content/PED_1_3X_Arsenic.asp?sitearea=PED. Accessed July 23, 2009.

14. National Cancer Institute. *Understanding Cancer and the Environment.* Available at www.cancer.gov/cancertopics/understandingcancer/environment. Accessed July 25, 2009.

15. American Cancer Society. *Benzene.* Available at www.cancer.org/docroot/ PED/content/PED_1_3X_Benzene.asp?sitearea=PED. Accessed July 23, 2009.

16. American Cancer Society. *Tetrachloroethylene. (Perchloroethylene).* Available at www.cancer.org/docroot/PED/content/PED_1_3x_Tetrachloroethylene_Perchloroethylene.asp?sitearea=PED. Accessed July 23, 2009.

17. US Environmental Protection Agency. *Frequently Asked Questions About Drycleaning.* Available at www.epa.gov/dfe/pubs/garment/ctsa/factsheet/ ctsafaq.htm. Accessed July 23, 2009.

18. National Institute of Environmental Health Sciences. *Endocrine Disruptors Fact Sheet,* June 2006.

19. National Cancer Institute. *Cancer Trends Progress Report—2007 Update. Pesticides.* Available at http://progressreport.cancer.gov/doc_detail.asp?pid= 1&did=2007&chid=71&coid=713&mid=. Accessed July 25, 2009/

20. Canadian Cancer Society. *Pesticide Exposure and Cancer.* Available at www.cancer.ca/Canada-wide/Prevention/Specific%20environmental%20 contaminants/Pesticides/Pesticide%20exposure%20and%20cancer.aspx?sc_ lang=en. Accessed July 25 2009.

21. American Cancer Society. *Cancer Facts and Figures 2004.* Available at www. cancer.org/downloads/STT/CAFF_finalPWSecured.pdf. Accessed December 22, 2009.

22. Bassil KL, Vakil C, Sanborn M, et al. Cancer health effects of pesticides. *Can Fam Phys.* 2007;53:1704–1711.

23. Alavanja MCR, Hoppin JA, Kamel F. Health effects of chronic pesticide exposure: cancer and neurotoxicity. *Ann Rev Public Health.* 2004;25:155–197.

24. American Cancer Society. *Common Questions About Diet and Cancer.* Available at www.cancer.org/docroot/PED/content/PED_3_2X_Common_Questions_About_Diet_and_Cancer.asp?sitearea=PED. Accessed July 25, 2009.

25. American Cancer Society. "Federal Report Looks at Risks from Plastics Chemical." ACS News Center, September 16, 2008. Available at www.cancer. org/docroot/NWS/content/NWS_1_1x_Federal_Report_Looks_at_Risks_ from_Plastics_Chemical.asp. Accessed July 25, 2009.

26. Parker-Pope T. "A Hard Plastic Is Raising Hard Questions." *New York Times*, April 22, 2008. Available at www.nytimes.com/2008/04/24/health/24iht-22-well.12301805.html?_r=1&scp=1&sq=a%20hard%20platic%20is%20raising%20hard%20questions&st=cse. Accessed July 25, 2009.

27. American Cancer Society. *Cellular Phones*. Available at www.cancer.org/docroot/PED/content/PED_1_3X_Cellular_Phones.asp. Accessed July 25, 2009.

28. American Cancer Society. *Cellular Phone Towers*. Available at www.cancer.org/docroot/PED/content/PED_1_3X_Cellular_Phone_Towers.asp?sitearea=PED. Accessed July 25, 2009.

29. American Cancer Society. *Hair Dyes*. Available at http://www.cancer.org/docroot/PED/content/PED_1_3X_Hair_Dye.asp?sitearea=PED. Accessed July 25, 2009.

30. American Cancer Society. *Radiation Exposure and Cancer*. Available at www.cancer.org/docroot/PED/content/PED_1_3X_Radiation_Exposure_and_Cancer.asp?sitearea=PED. Accessed July 25, 2009.

31. American Cancer Society. *Recombinant Bovine Growth Hormone*. Available at www.cancer.org/docroot/PED/content/PED_1_3x_Recombinant_Bovine_Growth_Hormone.asp. Accessed July 25, 2009.

32. American Cancer Society. *Water Fluoridation and Cancer Risk*. Available at www.cancer.org/docroot/PED/content/PED_1_3X_Water_Fluoridation_and_Cancer_Risk.asp?sitearea=PED. Accessed July 25, 2009.

33. US Department of Health and Human Services. *Cancer and the Environment. What Your Need to Know. What You Can Do*. Available at www.niehs.nih.gov/health/scied/documents/CancerEnvironment.pdf. Accessed July 25, 2009.

34. American Cancer Society. *Menopausal Hormone Replacement Therapy and Cancer Risk*. Available at www.cancer.org/docroot/CRI/content/CRI_2_6x_Menopausal_Hormone_Replacement_Therapy_and_Cancer_Risk.asp?sitearea=&level=. Accessed July 25, 2009.

35. Lichtenfeld L, American Cancer Society. *Dr. Len's Blog. How Dangerous Are CT Scans?* November, 29, 2007. Available at www.cancer.org/aspx/blog/Comments.aspx?id=180. Accessed July 25, 2009.

36. Brenner DJ, Hall EJ. Computed tomography—an increasing source of radiation exposure. *N Engl J Med*, 2007;357:2277–2284.

10

Making Decisions: Preventive Anticancer Medications and Surgeries

For many years, Barbara Pfeiffer thought that she and the women in her family were merely unlucky. Her mother and two of her aunts were diagnosed with breast cancer. She also knew that her grandmother probably had died of breast cancer before the age of 45. And 5 years after Barbara's mother was diagnosed with breast cancer, a second cancer developed in the other breast, and this time it was fatal.

Yet, when Barbara switched to a new gynecologist, her doctor encouraged her to *question* her family history of breast cancer. To her surprise, her doctor told her that because of her family history of cancer and her Ashkenazi Jewish heritage, she might be at risk for a hereditary breast cancer syndrome, likely owing to mutations (changes) in genes known as *BRCA1* or *BRCA2*. This inherited condition is thought to be responsible for between 5% and 10% of breast cancer cases. These gene mutations confer a greatly elevated risk not only of breast cancer but also of ovarian and other cancers.

Since Barbara had always been proactive about her health, she decided to undergo genetic counseling and testing and urged her mother to do the same. When they finally did get tested, they found that they both tested positive for the same *BRCA1* gene mutation. Her doctor immediately recommended an **oophorectomy**—in which the ovaries are removed—to reduce Barbara's risk of ovarian cancer. (According to studies, ovarian cancer risk is reduced by 85% to 95% by oophorectomy in hereditary breast and ovarian cancer syndromes but not completely eliminated because ovarian-like cancer can develop in tissue near the ovaries that is not removed.[1]) Studies also show that oopherectomy also reduces the risk of breast cancer by 50% to 60% for women with *BRCA* mutations when performed in women younger than age 50 (or before menopause).[6]

"At the time, he said, 'You can also have a preventive mastectomy,' but I dismissed it. I thought he was crazy," says Barbara now.

However, the *BRCA1* mutation confers up to an 85% risk of breast cancer, and although she was scheduled every 6 months for screening tests, Barbara found that she was living in fear. "I found that I was simply waiting for someone to tell me: *'You have breast cancer.'* It was incredibly stressful—for both me and my husband." So, in early 2005, Barbara decided on a choice that not many women make—a preventive mastectomy. Both her breasts were removed, and then, in the same operation, she underwent a breast reconstruction, in which the missing breast tissue was replaced by tissue from her abdomen. She also had a later operation to correct a complication—when blood flow to one of her new breasts was blocked by a twisted vein. Later that same year, in October 2005, her mother died of breast cancer.

Barbara's choice to have a preventive mastectomy reduced her risk for breast cancer by at least 90%. Yet it did not completely eliminate her risk because all the breast tissue cannot be completely removed in preventive mastectomy. So Barbara still needs regular exams and medical follow-up.[2]

Barbara says that she's glad she made the choice she did, but it definitely had an impact on her life. After the operations, she went through several months of recuperation. And there's no doubt about it—it was difficult to go through losing her natural breasts. "Sometimes I wish I looked the way I did before the surgeries," she says.

But the stress and anxiety she once associated with breast cancer are now gone, Barbara says. "At first it seemed to go against everything I've learned about health to remove healthy tissue to prevent a disease. But I'm happy with my decision. I no longer feel like a ticking time bomb—that breast cancer will be my future," she says.

Are Preventive Medications and Surgery Right for You?

Although you may not have a hereditary cancer syndrome like Barbara Pfeiffer, you may have wondered if preventive anticancer medications or surgery is a good choice for you. Perhaps you have a history of cancer in your family or a personal history of a precancerous condition that elevates your risk.

Before you jump to a decision about preventive medication or surgery, however, it's wise to find out if such a choice is appropriate for you and consider all the ramifications of your decision. This chapter will talk about the questions and issues you should consider—along with your doctor—if you are at higher risk than the average person and you are contemplating a choice for preventive medications or surgery. In this chapter you'll also find a discussion of the pros and cons of the most established preventive medications and operations for cancer, as well as some on the horizon.

On an intuitive level, preventive medication—and, to a lesser extent, preventive surgery—makes sense for those who are at high risk for developing cancer. Isn't it better to prevent cancer than to wait for a tumor to form and then treat it? Aren't your odds of surviving cancer better if you take a pill that reduces your risk rather than waiting for the disease to strike? Well, not always. The decision of whether or not to take a medication or have surgery to reduce your risk of cancer is not only an individual and personal choice but also a serious one. As Barbara Pfeiffer's story illustrates, there are inevitable tradeoffs one makes when one chooses to have a preventive operation or take preventive medication.

The term for taking medication to prevent cancer, as opposed to treating a malignancy after it develops, is **chemoprevention**. Several medications are now approved by the US Food and Drug Administration (FDA) to prevent breast and colon cancer for those at high risk,[8] and risk-reducing operations for cancer now include **mastectomy** and **oopherectomy.** Other surgeries for preventing cancer are **colectomy** (removal of the colon) for those with the inherited cancer syndrome known as *familial adenomatous polyposis* (FAP), who have a lifetime risk of colorectal cancer that is near 100%.[3] Removal of the thyroid for children who have the rare inherited familial medullary thyroid cancer syndrome can prevent a potentially fatal thyroid cancer from developing.[4] Those who have a rare mutation in a gene known as *CDH1*, which confers a high risk of stomach cancer, can have lifesaving surgery to remove their stomachs.[5]

Although preventive operations may seem drastic to most people, the concept of taking medication to prevent disease is not new. People at risk for heart attack are commonly prescribed baby aspirin or medications that treat hypertension or elevated cholesterol, which lower their heart attack risk. This approach has been accepted for years. Yet the choices involved in taking a preventive medication for cancer are more complicated because anticancer medications involve possible serious side effects as well as significant benefits for those at high risk.

Although research on chemoprevention has been ongoing since the early 1990s, the first chemopreventive agent to reach the clinic was **tamoxifen.** It was approved by the FDA as a risk-reduction medication for breast cancer in 1998 and has been shown to cut breast cancer incidence in high-risk women by 50%.[6] Tamoxifen was followed by **raloxifene (Evista)**, an osteoporosis drug that's been found to reduce breast cancer risk by 50% as well, and was approved by the FDA for breast cancer prevention in 2007.[7] **Finasteride** is another preventive cancer drug that has been found to cut prostate cancer risk by 25% to 30%.[8,9] **Celecoxib** is a drug that has been approved by the FDA for reducing polyp formation in people with FAP. People with FAP often have hundreds of polyps in the colon and rectum, and without treatment, these polyps can turn cancerous.[3]

However, the large-scale clinical trials that showed the benefits of these drugs for preventing cancer also brought to light serious side effects in some cases. This issue is a troublesome one when considering long-term administration of a drug to healthy people who may or may not develop cancer in the future.[10]

This is why it's important to note that most drugs for chemoprevention, such as tamoxifen, raloxifene, and celecoxib, are not recommended for those at average risk for cancer. They bring with them possible side effects, and all have both costs and benefits to consider. Since they are not risk-free, they're meant for people who are at elevated risk for the disease.

This is a key concept because many people overestimate their risk for cancer, particularly breast cancer. Knowing your true risk for cancer is vital in making a decision about preventive medications, surgery, or both. "Accurate risk assessment is an important cornerstone to decision making about prophylactic (preventive) medications or surgery," says Beth Peshkin, associate professor of oncology and senior genetic counselor at Georgetown's Lombardi Comprehensive Cancer Center. "It's also important to understand the potential risks and benefits of any therapy and its limitations."

Misperceptions about cancer risk are particularly problematic when it comes to breast cancer. Surveys have shown that up to 23% of women in the United States express interest in breast cancer chemoprevention based on their worry about the disease.[11,12] Fears about breast cancer tend to have a personal face—if you have a relative or friend who's had the disease or died from it, it's hard to dismiss the haunting quality of worries about it. But studies actually show that many women—including those who express an interest in breast cancer chemoprevention—may misperceive their risk for cancer and estimate their risk as much higher than it actually is. For instance, although surveys show that female smokers are nearly twice as likely as nonsmokers to express an interest in breast cancer chemoprevention,[12] the truth is that these women are much more at risk for heart attacks, stroke, and lung cancer. Smoking, however, has not been clearly linked to breast cancer risk.

So, given these misperceptions, as well as the significant downsides and benefits of anticancer medications and surgery, how can you make a good decision about these choices? Let's discuss the important issues to consider.[13-15]

Know Your Risk for Cancer

One of the most important steps you can take in deciding whether or not to take preventive medications or have preventive surgery is to get an accurate estimate of your risk for cancer. As mentioned in Chapter 3, if you have a strong family history of cancer, it is wise to go through an assessment of risk with a genetic counselor. You can find genetic counselors in your area through the National Cancer Institute Web site at www.cancer.gov/search/geneticsservices/.

There are also Web sites that provide assessments of your risk for different types of cancer based on questions you answer about your personal medical history, your family history of cancer, and your lifestyle. These Web sites include The Disease Risk Index from the Harvard School of Public Health and Your Disease Risk, a project of the Siteman Cancer Center at the Washington University School of Medicine (see "Resources" at the end of this chapter). At these sites, you can find out if your risk for cancer is low, average, or high.

If you think that you are at elevated risk for breast cancer, you also can try the risk assessment tools at the National Surgical Adjuvant Breast and Bowel Project or the National Cancer Institute's breast cancer risk assessment Web site (see "Resources" at the end of this chapter). They are based on the mathematical Gail model and provide numeric risk assessments showing your risk of getting breast cancer in 5 years and your risk of breast cancer throughout your lifetime. These tools can give you an idea if you are at above-average risk. A woman is considered at high risk for breast cancer and someone who might benefit from chemoprevention if her 5-year risk score is over 1.66%.

However, there's an important caution for using any of these Web sites: They should only be used along with a consultation with your doctor, who can explain the results to you more fully. One reason for this caution is that the online risk assessment tools have limitations, according to Peshkin. Some are devised according to the statistical Gail model, which considers only first-degree family history of breast cancer (in a mother, sister, or daughter). These models will underestimate risk for a woman who has a strong family history of breast cancer on her father's side (aunt or grandmother) and other second-degree relatives such as cousins. They are also not appropriate for those who've already had cancer.

Research the Options and Discuss Them With Your Physician

If you are at high risk, you will want to consider your options. In this case, knowledge is power. Have an in-depth discussion with your physician about what the alternatives are that can lower your risk. You also can find information about preventive cancer medications and operations at the American Cancer Society Web site at www.cancer.org and the National Cancer Institute Web site at www.nci.nih.gov.

Some Guidelines to Think About

In your conversations with your physician and your research, you'll want to think and talk about a range of issues. Some questions that you may want to ask yourself and that can help to guide you in your decision include the following.

How Much Does the Preventive Cancer Treatment Reduce My Risk?

Preventive anticancer medications such as tamoxifen, raloxifene, and finasteride can reduce risk by up to 30 to 50%, and preventive operations such as mastectomies can reduce the risk of breast cancer for high-risk women by up to 90% or more. But there are no absolute guarantees when it comes to preventing cancer. Every preventive anticancer therapy has limitations in reducing risk.

What Are the Possible Serious Side Effects of the Treatment or Medication?

In other words, does the treatment increase your risk of other serious medical conditions, such as stroke or heart disease, and how likely are you to suffer these side effects? In weighing the benefits and downsides of any anticancer medication or surgery, you'll want to consider your personal risk profile—are you more at risk for the cancer that the medication or operation prevents or for the complications it may cause? In coming up with this "personal risk profile," you'll want to contemplate factors such as your family medical history, your personal health history, your overall health, and your age.

If you are considering preventive surgery, you'll also want to think about the possible risk of complications. Every preventive surgery carries the risk of complications or even dying from surgery. Remember that your age and overall health affect your possible risk for complications.

Could Serious Side Effects Be Prevented or Lessened?

If the medication can cause serious side effects, it also helps to consider whether close monitoring by your physician and having regular screening tests could ease your fear of side effects.

What Are the Side Effects That Could Impact My Lifestyle?

Every medication or operation carries the chance for minor or major side effects, and you'll need to decide if these side effects are worth taking the medicine or undergoing the surgery. Although not everyone who takes a medication will experience side effects, there's a chance that you might. How much would these side effects affect your lifestyle?

In the case of preventive surgery, you're likely to have a recovery period that can last from several weeks to several months. How will you feel about going through such a recovery period? Could it hinder your lifestyle or your ability to make a living? You may have complications not only from the preventive surgery but also, as in the case of preventive mastectomy, from breast reconstruction. What might these complications be, and how likely are they to occur?

How Will the Therapy Affect My Self-image or My Sexuality?

Preventive surgery such as mastectomy will alter the way you look. Although plastic surgeons often can recreate the symmetry of the breast, the result may not be the same as your natural breasts. How will you feel about this outcome, and is your self-image strong enough to withstand a change in the way you look?

Some preventive medications also can change your ability to enjoy sex. Finasteride, which helps prevent prostate cancer, can cause sexual dysfunction in a small percentage of cases. Is the anticancer benefit worth this possible side effect?[16]

How Will My Decision Affect My Partner or Family?

Some preventive operations and medications can affect your sex life as well as your partner's sex life. Some also may impact your ability to have a family (as in the case of oophorectomy). How will your spouse or partner feel about these side effects? Is the reduction in cancer risk worth any sacrifices you may need to make in terms of sexuality or family? It's good to have an open discussion with your partner about your choice and how he or she feels about it.

What Is the Worst Possible Outcome, Whatever Your Decision?

To clarify your values, it often helps to consider the worst possible out-come of your decision. How would you feel if you decided not to take pre-ventive medication or have preventive surgery and you got breast cancer, ovarian cancer, or colon cancer several years down the line? Would the chance of suffering a serious side effect be worth the anticancer benefit of some medications or operations?

What Are the Other Alternatives to Reduce Risk?

If you are at increased risk of breast and colon cancer, there are some-times effective screening tools that can be used to catch precancerous conditions before they turn to cancer or to find cancer early when it is most treatable. For women at high risk of breast cancer, these screening tools (for finding early cancers) include **mammograms** and **magnetic resonance imaging (MRI)**. You should discuss the benefits and down-sides of each of these screening tools with your physician and which might be most suitable for you.

Consider the research about screening tools that prevent cancer. Some screening tools, such as **colonoscopy,** also have been shown to reduce incidence of colon cancer (by removing precancerous polyps) as well as being able to find cancer early. (For more on screening tools for cancer, see Chapter 8.) How comfortable do you feel relying on screenings to catch any possible cancer early? Remember that even the best screening tools some-times can miss cancer (called *false-negative results*) or indicate that you have cancer when the disease is not present (called *false-positive results*).

Lifestyle changes also could reduce your risk for cancer. Eating a healthy diet, attaining an appropriate weight, and regularly exercising can reduce cancer risk, most experts say. However, it's not known how much lifestyle changes can affect those who are at high genetic risk for cancer. Would you feel at ease with a decision to just make lifestyle changes to reduce your risk, and how likely are you to carry through on your intentions to maintain these lifestyle changes?

You also should consider if lifestyle changes are an appropriate pre-vention choice for *you.* For women at somewhat elevated risk for breast cancer because of family history, for instance, healthy lifestyle might reduce risk. Yet, for some inherited syndromes, such as FAP (which increases the risk for colon cancer) and familial medullary thyroid can-cer, lifestyle changes may not affect risk much or even at all. Certainly, making lifestyle changes that confer other health benefits aside from can-cer risk reduction may be valuable. They may reduce your risk for other diseases, such as heart disease or diabetes. And it's one aspect of your healthcare that you can control, and therefore, it can be psychologically beneficial and empowering.

How Distressed Are You About Your Cancer Risk?

Although there are many factors to consider when making a decision about preventive medication or surgery, the bottom line is that every decision is a personal one. How anxious and stressed are you about your risk for cancer? If your stress level is high and your actual risk is high as well, then you may want to consider discussing anticancer medications or surgery with your physician. According to a number of scientific research studies, worry about breast cancer is often a key predictor of choosing interventions such as preventive mastectomy.[13–15]

Consider how your decision—whether it's for or against preventive medications or surgery—will affect your stress and anxiety level.

Summing It Up: Questions to Consider About Preventive Therapies

- What is my actual risk, and is it high enough to merit anticancer therapy?

- How much will the treatment or surgery reduce my risk?

- What are the possible serious side effects of treatment?

- What side effects might impact my lifestyle and comfort level?

- How will the decision affect my sexuality or self-image?

- How will my partner react, and will the treatment affect my ability to have a family?

- What are the most extreme outcomes of my decision?

- Are there other alternatives to reduce risk, and how effective are they?

- Will the treatment or therapy reduce my distress level about cancer?

In addition to the physical consequences of your decision, you'll want to consider the psychological and emotional results as well.

The rest of this chapter is devoted to a brief discussion of several preventive anticancer therapies now in use. It also will delve into some recent clinical trials of new or promising anticancer medications. Remember that if you are considering anticancer therapy, an in-depth discussion with your healthcare provider should be your first step.

Tamoxifen and Raloxifene: Two Drugs for Preventing Breast Cancer

Tamoxifen and **raloxifene** are two drugs that are similar in many ways.[10] They both help to prevent breast cancer in women at high risk. Their method of action is much the same—these two drugs interfere with the action of the hormone estrogen, which can fuel the growth of breast cancer cells. They also can help to prevent **osteoporosis,** or weakening of the bones, in women after menopause. For many years, tamoxifen has been used as a treatment for breast cancer and to stop breast cancer from coming back in women who have already had the disease. Raloxifene (Evista) has been used widely as a treatment for osteoporosis.

There are some significant benefits to taking tamoxifen and raloxifene as well as some possible serious side effects.

Benefits of Tamoxifen

- Reduces the risk of invasive breast cancer by about half
- Reduces the risk of noninvasive breast cancer, such as ductal carcinoma in situ in which cancer is confined to the milk ducts of the breast, by one-third
- Helps to prevent osteoporosis and reduces the risk of bone fracture of the hip, wrist, and spine by one-third

Tamoxifen is a powerful therapy. In addition to preventing breast cancer and osteoporosis, it can increase the risk of some rare but serious health problems, including

- Endometrial cancer (cancer of the lining of the uterus)
- Uterine sarcoma (cancer of the connective tissue of the uterus)
- Major blood clots (pulmonary embolism or blood clot in the lung, stroke, and deep vein thrombosis or the formation of a blood clot deep within the body, usually in a leg vein)
- Cataracts

Side effects of tamoxifen can include hot flashes, vaginal dryness, depression, loss of appetite, nausea, dizziness, headaches, weight gain, and fatigue. However, there are treatments that can eliminate or reduce many of these side effects—and many of these side effects are quite rare.

In the clinical trial known as the Study of Tamoxifen and Raloxifene (STAR), the benefits and side effects of tamoxifen and raloxifene were compared. The scientists found that tamoxifen and raloxifene both reduced the risk of invasive breast cancer by about 50%. Women taking raloxifine were more likely than those taking tamoxifen to develop noninvasive breast cancer (such as cancer confined to the milk ducts). However, the difference between the two drugs in preventing noninvasive breast cancer could have been due to chance and more research is needed to resolve this question.

While raloxifene can cause side effects, there may be less risk of serious side effects than with tamoxifen. Raloxifene can cause blood clots in the legs or lungs, however, in the STAR trial, women taking raloxifene had 30% fewer blood clots than those on tamoxifen. It's not clear if raloxifene increases the risk of uterine cancer, but if it does, this increase may be less than that seen with tamoxifen. The risks of cataracts and stroke seem to be less likely in women who take raloxifene versus those who take tamoxifen. Serious side effects for both drugs seem to occur less often in those under age 50 than in older women, according to recent guidelines from the American Society of Clinical Oncology.[17]

Side effects of raloxifene include

- Hot flashes
- Vaginal dryness or irritation
- Leg cramps
- Flulike symptoms
- Joint pain[7]
- Swelling in the hands and feet

Both tamoxifen and raloxifene are usually taken for a course of 5 years. When taken for 5 years, they seem to reduce the risk of breast cancer for at least 10 years, according to the guidelines from the American Society of Clinical Oncology.[17] Women also should not get pregnant when on these preventive breast cancer medications because they can cause harm to developing embryos.

Tamoxifen is approved for use in women who are at high risk for breast cancer who are premenopausal or postmenopausal (having gone through menopause). Women at high risk for breast cancer can include those with genetic breast cancer syndromes, as well as women with a very strong family history of the disease, and those who've had a precancerous or cancerous condition that increased their risk for breast cancer. Raloxifene is approved only for high-risk women after menopause.

Who Should Take Tamoxifen and Raloxifene?

These medications are appropriate only for women who have a Gail risk score of at least 1.66. The Gail model estimates a woman's risk for breast cancer. The Gail risk score is derived from a series of questions about factors that can increase breast cancer risk. Some women who might receive benefit from these drugs include

- Women with a mutation in the *BRCA1* or *BRCA2* genes or with a hereditary risk of breast cancer, although studies on this population are limited
- Women who've had a breast biopsy that showed precancerous or cancerous conditions that increase their risk of invasive breast cancer, called *atypical ductal hyperplasia* or *lobular carcinoma in situ*
- A strong family history of breast cancer—that is, several close relatives with the disease, especially if it was diagnosed before menopause
- Women whose age, reproductive history, or family history of breast cancer (or a combination thereof) confer an elevated risk the disease

Are There Women Who Should Not Take These Medicines?

Women who should be cautious about taking these medicines for preventing breast cancer, particularly tamoxifen, include

- Women who have a history of blood clots
- Those who take a medicine to thin their blood
- Those who have a history of high blood pressure, smoking, obesity, or diabetes
- Women planning to become pregnant or who are pregnant
- Women who have not had breast cancer risk assessment
- Those who are not at increased risk for breast cancer
- Women currently taking hormone-replacement therapy

For more detailed information on tamoxifen and raloxifene, see the American Cancer Society Web site and the fact sheet entitled, *Medicines to Reduce Breast Cancer Risk*, available at the American Cancer Society Web site.

On the Horizon: A New Preventive Therapy for Breast Cancer

Aromatase inhibitors are drugs that are sometimes used to treat advanced breast cancer or to prevent breast cancer from returning in those who have been diagnosed with the disease. These drugs include **exemestane (Aromasin), anastrozole (Arimidex),** and **letrozole (Femara).**[10] Unlike tamoxifen and raloxifene, these drugs have not been approved by the FDA for preventing breast cancer in high-risk women. However, studies are now underway to see if these medications can reduce breast cancer risk in women who have not been diagnosed with the disease.[10]

Side effects of these drugs include joint stiffness and pain, similar to having arthritis in different joints at the same time. However, aromatase inhibitors are less likely than tamoxifen to cause serious blood clots and do not seem to raise the risk of endometrial cancer or uterine sarcoma. However, unlike tamoxifen and raloxifene, these drugs actually increase the risk of bone fractures and speed up the bone-thinning process that can happen after menopause. Because these drugs are newer than raloxifene and tamoxifen, less is known about their long-term side effects. Currently, they're not recommended for breast cancer risk prevention outside clinical trials.[17,18]

Preventive Mastectomy

Preventive mastectomy is the surgical removal of one or both breasts to prevent breast cancer. There are two types of preventive mastectomy: total or subcutaneous mastectomy. In a **total mastectomy,** the doctor removes the entire breast and nipple. In some types of total mastectomy, however, the skin is spared. In **subcutaneous mastectomy,** the nipple and areola (the colored skin surrounding the nipple) are left intact to preserve appearance and nipple sensation. Some tissue remains under the areola after subcutaneous mastectomy. It is generally believed that a total mastectomy provides the most protection against breast cancer.[19]

Women who are at high risk of developing breast cancer might consider undergoing preventive mastectomy. According to guidelines issued by the Society of Surgical Oncology and information from the National Cancer Institute, these risks include[19,20]

- *BRCA1 or BRCA2 mutations*—A woman who tests positive for either of these two breast cancer gene mutations has a high risk of developing breast cancer.
- *Family history of breast cancer*—Some women, even those without a known *BRCA1* or *BRCA2* mutation, may have a very strong history of breast cancer, in which breast cancer was diagnosed in multiple relatives before age 50. If a woman's relative or relatives were diagnosed with both breast and ovarian cancer, her risk for breast cancer may be even higher.
- *Previous breast cancer*—Some women who have had cancer in one breast may be more likely to develop a new cancer in the opposite breast, particularly if they have other risk factors as well. A preventive mastectomy for the opposite breast might be considered in cases where there's a known *BRCA1* or *BRCA2* mutation, a strong history of breast cancer in multiple family members, or known abnormal changes in the breast (see below).
- A *previous biopsy showing abnormal changes in the breast*— These changes include atypical ductal or lobular hyperplasia or lobular carcinoma in situ and indicate increased breast cancer risk. These changes are particularly significant if a woman also has a strong family history of breast cancer, and in rare cases, preventive mastectomy may be considered.
- *Diffuse and indeterminate breast microcalcifactions or dense breasts*—In rare cases, a preventive mastectomy might be considered for a woman who has breast microcalcifications (tiny deposits of calcium in the breast) or dense breast tissue, both of which are linked to an increased risk of breast cancer as well as difficulties in diagnosing abnormalities.
- *Radiation therapy*—In rare cases, mastectomy might be considered for a woman who has had radiation to the chest (including the breast) before age 30 (usually to treat Hodgkin lymphoma) because such women have increased risk for breast cancer. A preventive mastectomy might be considered in these women if they also have other risk factors.

It is important for any woman considering preventive mastectomy to talk with her doctor about the procedure and her risk of developing cancer, as well as the role of genetic testing in clarifying risks. She also should discuss possible complications, including any complications from breast reconstruction surgery. Her decision should be considered in the light of her individual risk factors and her level of concern about breast cancer. Complications from preventive mastectomy and reconstruction include infection and bleeding, movement of the implant, and contracture (the formation of scar tissue around the implant) in some cases.[19] Although preventive mastectomy can reduce the risk of breast cancer significantly (by about 90% or more), it cannot totally protect against the disease. Breast tissue is widely distributed on the chest wall and sometimes can be found in the armpit and close to the collarbone—making it difficult for the surgeon to remove all breast tissue. After preventive mastectomy, a woman still will need to be monitored by her physician with follow-up care and regular breast exams.[19]

In addition to possible complications, the drawbacks of preventive mastectomy include psychological effects. Some women may experience changes in self-esteem and self-image after a preventive mastectomy.[19] This is why discussing your feelings about this procedure with your clinician—if you're considering it—is important. You also can ask if your doctor can introduce you to women who've had preventive mastectomies to get an idea of what it is like to go through this procedure. You also can contact the organization Facing Our Risk of Cancer Empowered (FORCE), which provides peer support and information for women with hereditary breast cancer (see "Resources" below).

Many women choose to have breast reconstruction after a preventive mastectomy—either at the time of the mastectomy or at a time following the initial operation. If you're considering breast reconstruction and are discussing this option with a plastic surgeon, you can ask to see the results of plastic surgery to get an idea of how your breasts will look afterward. Many plastic surgeons keep a "scrapbook" of results of their procedures.

In breast reconstruction, the plastic surgeon may insert an implant (a balloon-like device filled with silicone or saline) under the skin and chest muscles. Another procedure, called **autologous tissue reconstruction,** uses fat, muscle, and skin from the woman's buttocks, back, or abdomen to create the breast shape. Reconstruction with implants usually requires less surgery and often is recommended for those over 65 years of age or those who are not in good physical condition and might have difficulty tolerating a longer operation. However, with an implant, there's a risk of capsular contracture (formation of scar tissue around the implant), which makes the reconstructed breast feel unnaturally hard and also can be painful. Breast reconstruction done with tissue-flap reconstruction has the advantage of creating a softer, more natural breast. An implant generally will look and feel worse with time, but breasts reconstructed with autologous tissue often improve. They often feel, move, and look like a real breast.[21]

In addition to considering the results of plastic surgery, you also should ask what kind of follow-up care you should receive after preventive mastectomy or breast reconstruction. Some women who have breast reconstruction using tissue from their abdomen, back, or buttocks may have exercise limitations after surgery and/or may need physical therapy afterward.[19]

Oophorectomy: Preventing Cancer by Surgically Removing Your Ovaries

If you are a carrier of either the *BRCA1* or *BRCA2* gene mutation, one option to reduce your risk of both breast and ovarian cancer is an **oophorectomy,** in which both your ovaries are removed. Preventive oophorectomy is considered one of the most effective means of preventing ovarian cancer in women with a *BRCA* mutation; in most of these women, the fallopian tubes should be removed along with the ovaries to decrease the risk of cancer. This procedure is called a **salpingo-oophorectomy.**[1]

Your ovaries hold eggs, control your reproductive cycle, and secrete hormones.

Removing your ovaries greatly decreases the secretion of the hormones progesterone and estrogen, which also can slow down or halt breast cancer development and growth.[23] A recent analysis of 10 independent scientific studies showed that salpingo-oophorectomy can reduce risk for both ovarian or fallopian tube cancer by 80% and risk for breast cancer by 50% in those with a genetic breast and ovarian cancer syndrome.[22]

For high-risk women (those with a mutation in the *BRCA1* or *BRCA2* gene), oophorectomy may be a good choice because there are few good screening options for ovarian cancer. Unlike breast cancer, it is difficult to catch ovarian cancer at an early stage. Most women with ovarian cancer are diagnosed at a late stage, and thus the survival rates from this cancer are low. (For more on ovarian cancer screening, see Chapter 8.)

Oophorectomy brings on early menopause when it is performed in younger women. If you decide to undergo oophorectomy, you'll need to understand the risks and results of the surgery. After oophorectomy, you'll lose the ability to have children. Other risks include[23]

- *Osteoporosis*—If you have your ovaries removed when you are premenopausal, the surgery can bring on early menopause, which reduces the bone-protecting effects of estrogen. As a result, you'll be at increased risk for the bone-thinning disease osteoporosis and increased risk of fractures.[23]

- *Menopausal symptoms*—Early menopause can cause symptoms such as hot flashes, sexual problems, vaginal dryness, and insomnia. In most women, these symptoms are only mildly uncomfortable; however, if they disrupt your daily life, treatments are available.[23]
- *Cancer*—Preventive oophorectomy reduces the risk of cancer but doesn't completely eliminate it. Although it can reduce the risk for ovarian cancer substantially, there is a slight chance of a type of cancer that affects the peritoneum, the lining of the abdomen.[1]

Aside from being a *BRCA* carrier, other women who might consider preventive oophorectomy include those with a personal or strong family history of breast cancer (in first degree relatives) before menopause or age 50 and those with one or more close family members diagnosed with ovarian cancer. If you think that you are at high risk for ovarian cancer or might have a *BRCA* mutation, it's important to make an appointment to see a genetic counselor. The genetic counselor can help you to assess your cancer risk, discuss whether or not you should undergo genetic testing, and provide guidance in your decisions about preventive surgery.[23]

Protecting Against Colon Cancer: The Pros and Cons of COX-2 Inhibitors

Celecoxib—and other drugs known as **COX-2 inhibitors**—have been shown to significantly reduce precancerous colon growths that can lead to colon cancer, according to recent studies. These drugs reduce inflammation in the body and are sometimes used to treat arthritis. They block an enzyme called *cyclooxygenase-2* (COX-2), which is overproduced when tissues are inflamed. And their use seems to reduce the dangerous precancerous colon growths called *adenomas* that can lead to colon cancer. However, there's a serious downside to these drugs. Studies have found that as well as decreasing colon cancer risk, these drugs increase the risk of heart disease.

Although COX-2 inhibitors are being studied for their possible role in preventing cancer in people at high risk of colon cancer, they aren't recommended for widespread use.[24] However, celecoxib has been approved by the FDA for use as chemoprevention in people who have the hereditary condition FAP, in which hundreds of precancerous polyps form in the colon and rectum. Untreated, this inherited condition almost invaria-bly leads to colon cancer. The drug is used primarily—along with surgery that removes the colon—to prevent polyps in the rectum that remains.[25]

Researchers are now working to understand why COX-2 inhibitors increase the risk for cardiovascular disease and are attempting to iden-tify **biologic markers**—or chemical markers in our bodies—that might indicate which people are more likely to benefit from these medicines and less likely to have side effects.[24]

On the Horizon: a New Drug Combo Lowers Colon Cancer Risk

In April 2008, researchers showed for the first time that a com-bination of the drug **difluoromethylornithine (DFMO)**, usually used to treat advanced cancers, and a **nonsteroi-dal anti-inflammatory drug (NSAID)** called **sulindac (Clinoril)** reduces the risk of recurrent colorectal adenomas by up to 95%.[26] Adenomas are growths that are likely to turn into colorectal cancer. NSAIDs are drugs that reduce swelling and inflammation and are used commonly to treat arthritis.

The study treated 375 patients who had a history of at least one colorectal polyp with either DFMO and sulindac or placebo (a "sugar pill"). The DFMO dose used was about 1/50 the strength of that used to treat advanced cancer. In addition to being effective in reducing precancerous colon growth, the drug combination produced no significant side effects.

Further studies will research the two drugs in combina-tion and at different doses to further test their effectiveness and safety. They are not presently approved for the preven-tion of colorectal cancer, even in high-risk patients.

Finasteride: A Medication That Lowers Prostate Cancer Risk

When the medication **finasteride** was first studied as a possible means of lowering prostate cancer risk, scientific findings were mixed. A large clin-ical trial of nearly 19,000 men, followed for 7 years, found that finasteride reduced prostate cancer risk by 25%. However, it also seemed to increase the risk for developing high-grade prostate tumors, or tumors that are more likely to grow and spread. And the tumors it prevented seemed to be so slow growing that they posed little risk to patients.[8]

Yet a new analysis of the data, released in May 2008, showed that fin-asteride reduced prostate cancer even more than previously thought—by

25% to 30%—and did not increase the risk of more aggressive cancer. In fact, the new analysis showed that finasteride actually decreased the rate of aggressive tumors by 28%. And most of the tumors prevented were those that could spread and cause death.[8]

Finasteride is approved by the FDA for treating *benign prostatic hyperplasia* (BPH, enlargement of the prostate) in low doses and for treating prostate cancer in higher doses. It is also used as a treatment for male baldness. The dosage used in the prevention trial of finasteride was the same as that used to treat BPH.

Side effects of finasteride include erectile dysfunction and lowered sexual desire. However, in clinical trials it seemed to help with urinary problems such as trouble urinating and leaking urine (incontinence).[16]

In recently published guidelines, the American Society of Clinical Oncology and the American Urological Association recommended that men who undergo regular prostate-specific antigen (PSA) screening, have a PSA ≤3.0 ng/mL, and are without symptoms of prostate cancer could benefit from a discussion about the benefits and risks of taking finasteride. The benefits of finasteride include significant reduction in prostate cancer risk and a 50% reduction in PSA within 12 months. The possible risks include the possibility of high-grade prostate cancer and side effects such as erectile dysfunction.[27] Men who have BPH or those with a family history or other risk factors for prostate cancer also should consider talking with their physicians about using finasteride either to treat BPH or for cancer prevention. BPH is considered a noncancerous enlargement of the prostate but does not increase prostate cancer risk.[8]

Resources

To find out more about assessing your risk for cancer, you can visit the following Web sites. These Web sites should be used only in consultation with your clinician.

The Disease Risk Index from the Harvard School of Public Health
www.diseaseriskindex.harvard.edu/update/
Your Disease Risk
www.yourdiseaserisk.wustl.edu/

To assess your risk for breast cancer, you can try these Web sites
National Surgical Adjuvant Breast and Bowel Project
www.breastcancerprevention.org
National Cancer Institute breast cancer risk assessment tool
www.cancer.gov/bcrisktool/

If you'd like more information about hereditary breast or ovarian cancer and preventive treatment approaches, you can visit the Web site of FORCE at www.facingourrisk.org/.

References

1. American Cancer Society. *Can Ovarian Cancer Be Prevented?* Available at www.cancer.org/docroot/CRI/content/CRI_2_4_2X_Can_ovarian_cancer_be_prevented_33.asp?sitearea=. Accessed July 28,2009.

2. American Cancer Society. *Can Breast Cancer Be Prevented?* Available at www.cancer.org/docroot/CRI/content/CRI_2_4_2X_Can_breast_cancer_be_prevented_5.asp?rnav=cri. Accessed July 28, 2009.

3. American Cancer Society. *Can Colorectal Cancer Be Prevented?* Available at www.cancer.org/docroot/CRI/content/CRI_2_4_2X_Can_colon_and_rectum_cancer_be_prevented.asp?sitearea=. Accessed July 28, 2009.

4. American Cancer Society. *Can Thyroid Cancer Be Prevented?* Available at www.cancer.org/docroot/CRI/content/CRI_2_4_2X_Can_thyroid_cancer_be_prevented_43.asp?sitearea=. Accessed July 28, 2009.

5. American Cancer Society. *Inherited Stomach Cancer Is Prevented with Surgery.* Available at www.cancer.org/docroot/NWS/content/update/NWS_1_1xU_Inherited_Stomach_Cancer_Is_Prevented_With_Surgery.asp. Accessed July 28, 2009.

6. Lichtenfed L, American Cancer Society. *Dr. Len's Cancer Blog. A New Era for Breast Cancer Prevention*, April 17, 2006. Available at www.cancer.org/aspx/blog/Comments.aspx?id=69. Accessed July 28, 2009.

7. US Food and Drug Administration. *FDA Approves New Uses for Evista*, September 17, 2007. Available at www.fda.gov/NewsEvents/Newsroom/PressAnnouncements/2007/ucm108981.htm. Accessed July 30, 2009.

8. National Cancer Institute. *Studies Make Case for Finasteride to Prevent Prostate Cancer.* Available at www.cancer.gov/clinicaltrials/results/PCPT0608. Accessed July 30, 2009.

9. "Finasteride May Help Prevent Development of Prostate Cancer, Study Shows." *Science Daily*, May 20, 2008.

10. American Cancer Society. *Medicines to Reduce Breast Cancer Risk.* Available at www.cancer.org/docroot/CRI/content/CRI_2_6X_Tamoxifen_and_Raloxifene_Questions_and_Answers_5.asp. Accessed July 28, 2009.

11. Bastian LA, Lipkus IM, Kuchibhatla MN, et al.Women's interest in chemoprevention for breast cancer. *Arch Intern Med.* 2001;161:1639–1644.

12. Mulley AG, Sepucha K. Making good decisions about breast cancer chemoprevention. *Ann Intern Med.* 2002;137:52–54.

13. Stefanek M, Hartmann L, Nelson W, et al. Risk-reduction mastectomy: clinical issues and research needs. *J Natl Cancer Inst.* 2001;93:1297–306.

14. Stefanek M, Enger C, Benkendorf J, et al. Bilateral prophylactic mastectomy decision making: a vignette study. *Prev Med.* 1999;29:216–221.

15. Stefanek M, Helzlsouer, Wilcox PM, et al. Predictor of and satisfaction with bilateral prophylactic mastectomy. *Prev Med.* 1995;24:412–419.

16. American Cancer Society. *Can Prostate Cancer Be Prevented?* Available at www.cancer.org/docroot/CRI/content/CRI_2_4_2X_Can_prostate_cancer_be_prevented_36.asp?sitearea=. Accessed July 28, 2009.

17. Visvanathan K, Chlebowski RT, Hurley P, et al. American Society of Clinical Oncology practice guideline update on the use of pharmacologic interventions including tamoxifen, raloxifene and aromatase inhibition for breast cancer risk reduction. *J Clin Oncol.* 2009; 27:3235–3258.

18. American Cancer Society. *Detailed Guide—Breast Cancer. Hormone Therapy.* Available at www.cancer.org/docroot/CRI/content/CRI_2_4_4X_Hormone_Therapy_5.asp?sitearea=. Accessed July 30, 2009.

19. National Cancer Institute. *Preventive Mastectomy: Questions and Answers.* Available at www.cancer.gov/cancertopics/factsheet/Therapy/preventive-mastectomy. Accessed July 30, 2009.

20. Society of Surgical Oncology. *Statement on Prophylactic Mastectomy,* March 2007. Available at www.surgonc.org/default.aspx?id=47. Accessed July 30, 2009.

21. MD Anderson.org. *Breast Reconstruction.* Available at www3.mdanderson.org/DEPARTMENTS/plastic/ptbreast.htm. Accessed July 30, 2009.

22. National Cancer Institute. *Removal of Ovaries and Fallopian Tubes Cuts Cancer Risk for BRCA 1 and BRCA2 Carriers.* Available at www.cancer.gov/clinicaltrials/results/BRCA0209. Accessed July 30, 2009.

23. MayoClinic.com. *Prophylactic Oophorectomy: Preventing Cancer by Surgically Removing Your Ovaries.* Available at www.mayoclinic.com/health/breast-cancer/WO00095. Accessed July 30, 2009.

24. Lockmuller J. National Institutes of Health. *Colorectal Cancer Fact Sheet,* September 2007.

25. Wehbi M, Griglione NM, Yang VW, et al. Emedicine. Medscape.com. *Familial Adenomatous Polyposis: Treatment & Medication.* Available at http://emedicine.medscape.com/article/175377-treatment. Accessed July 30, 2009.

26. American Association for Cancer Research. "Low Dose DFMO Reduces Colon Cancer Risk Without Toxicity," news release, April 14, 2008. Available at www.aacr.org/home/public—media/aacr-press-releases/press-releases-2008.aspx?d=1046. Accessed July 30, 2009.

27. Kramer BS, Hagerty KL, Justman S, et al. Use of 5-alpha-reductase inhibitors for prostate cancer chemoprevention: American Society of Clinical Oncology/American Urological Association 2008 clinical practice guideline. J Clin Oncol. 2009;27:1502–1516.

11

When You've Already Had Cancer: Steps You Can Take for Good Health

"Cancer is like a giant magnifying glass," says John (not his real name), a prostate cancer survivor. "When you're standing in the shadow of cancer, it magnifies the good things in life and gives clarity to the things that aren't so good."

"But cancer has given me a chance to view the glass as half full—something I'd like to think I've been mostly successful at," John adds. Part of John's journey in "seeing the glass half full" after his diagnosis and treatment for prostate cancer was to start a support group for younger men diagnosed with prostate cancer at the Markstein Cancer Education Center and Prevention Services at Alta Bates Medical Center, near San Francisco. Called "PC in the City," the group is meant to give younger men a place to talk about their struggles with cancer, as well as the aftereffects of treatment.

"Prostate cancer can be an entirely different disease for a younger man that it is for one who is older. *Developing prostate cancer at a younger age adds layers of complexity—because younger men may still want to have a family; have parents, grandparents, [and] burgeoning careers; and may* be more concerned about sexual potency," he says (erectile dysfunction can be a side effect of prostate cancer treatment).

As the leader of PC in the City, John helps new members of the support group navigate through the difficulties of being a cancer patient and then being a cancer survivor. "There's a lot of sharing about intimate things that goes on in the group—but at the same time, it's pretty dignified," he says.

Another cancer survivor who has found help through a support group at the Markstein Cancer Education Center is Douglas Beckstein, who was diagnosed with stage III colon cancer in 2003. For several years he's been attending a twice-monthly writing group made up of cancer survivors called "In Other Words." "The main thing you get from writing about your experience with cancer is that it helps you release your feelings and tell your story. And because other cancer survivors are in the group, you find a sense of community," he says. Writing has been very helpful in the emotional healing process after cancer, he adds.

Like many survivors, Doug's encounter with cancer was life-changing. "It was like dying and coming back to life. I really began to appreciate when I could walk, climb stairs, hike, and ride a bicycle again after cancer treatments," says Doug, who is now cancer-free.

As a result of his cancer diagnosis, Doug has made a point of living as healthy a life as possible. His tips for healthy living are to manage stress, get enough sleep, and eat a healthy diet. Avid about exercise, he also maintains an extensive network of supportive friends and has made having fun a priority. "My calendar is filled with fun things to do—every day. After I came through cancer, I decided that I was going to have a vibrant, rich life, and I was going to enjoy each day," he says.

John's and Doug's experiences echo those of many cancer survivors. After being diagnosed with cancer and going through treatment, it's not unusual for people to change their lifestyle to bring more personal meaning into their lives. Their health concerns are also similar to those of other survivors. After a bout with cancer, it's possible that you'll need to deal with aftereffects of treatment that may impact your health, such as increased risk for heart disease, diabetes, and osteoporosis. Many survivors are also concerned about recurrence—or the chance that the cancer may return—and want to know what steps to take to best reduce their risk of the disease recurring.

This chapter is meant to address the concerns of cancer survivors—particularly when it comes to reducing the risk of recurrence or second cancers—steps that can help you to be as healthy as possible following treatment. Although ending treatment is a just cause for celebration for many survivors—there are also health issues that are likely to persist. This chapter also will talk about the understandable fears of recurrence that trouble many survivors and lifestyle changes and other measures that may help you to reduce your risk.

More than 11 million people in the United States are cancer survivors.[1] The growing number of cancer survivors reflects some amazing medical advances, including better detection and new, more effective treatments. You should know that many survivors go on to lead long and healthy lives after diagnosis and treatment. As with everything else in life, though, there are no guarantees. As a survivor, you're also more at risk for cancer than the average person. There is a chance that your cancer can recur, or come back, or that a second cancer can develop. In fact, cancer survivors have about a 14% higher risk than does the general population of developing a new cancer, according to a National Cancer Institute report based on data from 1973 to 2000.[2]

What does this mean for you? After treatment, many survivors want to know what the risk is for their cancer to recur. In many ways, however, what survivors may be looking for is reassurance. They don't want to be afraid that their cancer will come back, and, in fact, they'd like to know that they're "cured" and that the cancer will not recur.

Unfortunately, whether or not your cancer will recur is sometimes hard to predict. It also can depend on the type of cancer you had, its initial stage, and the type of treatment. Although treatment methods can make a difference in many cancers, they are not perfect. Sometimes small clusters of cancer cells too small to be found on imaging scans may remain and then grow and spread. Other times the cancer is very aggressive, and even chemotherapy or radiation may not have killed all the cancer cells because some of them could be resistant to those treatments. On the other hand, you could survive for many years after cancer treatment, and cancer may never trouble you again.

If you're afraid about the possibility that your cancer may recur, you're not alone. Many cancer survivors—about 70%—report significant concern that their cancer may recur, according to the American Cancer Society.[3] You may want to put the experience of cancer behind you, but fears about it may worry you. These fears even may make it difficult to sleep, be close to your partner, or make decisions. To some degree, this is entirely normal, and it's a process that many survivors go through after treatment. The good news is that, as more time passes, the less likely these fears are to trouble you. However, if these anxieties start to interfere with your life, then it may be time to seek help from a therapist, psychologist, or other mental health professional.[3]

You should know that recurrence of cancer can happen, and you should consider having an open and honest discussion with your physician about this fact. He or she can help you to understand your risk—or the chances that your cancer will recur—given the type of cancer you had, how aggressive it was, and what kind of treatment you received. Although this discussion may be unsettling in some cases and reassuring in others, it can help you to understand your risk of recurrence. Then you can talk with your physician about the best ways to reduce your risk.

It's important to note that although there may be some things you can do that can help to reduce your risk of cancer recurrence or a second

cancer, there is no absolute guarantee. Neither is there any magic supplement or lifestyle change that will guarantee that your cancer will not
recur or that a second cancer will not occur.

When my father was diagnosed with lung cancer, I was well aware
of the dire statistics for this type of cancer. Not many people with lung
cancer survive for 5 years. However, after treatment, my father went on
to develop a healthy happy lifestyle. He gave up smoking for good, walked
2 miles every day, and took up regular golfing with his neighborhood bud-
dies. When 5 years had passed after my father's operation for lung cancer,
my brother and I breathed a sigh of relief. We thought my father was one
of the lucky ones.

Unfortunately, several months after a fall on the ice outside his Long
Island home, the cause of a new chest pain was discovered. It was lung
cancer, and this time it had spread to his bones. The diagnosis was not
good. In fact, in our first session with his oncologist, we talked merely
about ways to make my father comfortable. There was no hope of remis-
sion. His oncologist told us that my father's lung cancer probably was a
second cancer rather than a recurrence. Because my father was a former
heavy smoker, his lungs had sustained enough damage for a second cancer to grow.

Was there something my father could have done to stop his second
cancer from invading his lungs and his bones? Probably not. And that's a
truth that's sometimes hard to accept. If you're a cancer survivor, there is
really nothing you can do that can provide absolute reassurance that your
cancer *definitely* will not come back. Sometimes life just doesn't play fair.

That said, however, there are some measures you can take that scientific studies show may help to *reduce your risk* of your cancer recurring
or a second cancer from taking hold. These health measures—such as not
smoking and losing weight if you are overweight—also will help to protect
you against other health problems, such as heart disease and diabetes.

First, one of the most important steps you can take is to have a
discussion with your doctor about your risk and what measures she or
he thinks will help you to be as healthy as possible. Learning what you
can do for your health not only will keep you as healthy as possible, both
physically and psychologically, but also can give you a feeling of control.

Healthcare After Cancer

To be as healthy as possible as a cancer survivor, the first step you should
take after treatment is to come up with a "survivorship care plan."[4-6] This
is a comprehensive plan for your healthcare devised by you and your
clinician. (For information on survivor care plans and other aspects of

The Emotions of Cancer: Dealing With Fears of Recurrence

Fears that your cancer might recur are entirely normal and trouble many survivors. Here are a few suggestions to ease those fears[4]:

- Be aware that you don't have control over some aspects of your cancer. Accepting this thought is one way to ease your emotions.

- Express your feelings of fear with a trusted friend or counselor. Being open about your fears may help you to feel less worried.

- Observe your fearful thoughts—but don't judge them. Practice letting them go. Some people picture their worries floating away or turn to a higher power for help in handling them.

- Try to live in the present moment rather than worrying about the future or dwelling in the past. If there's a way you can find to be at peace within yourself, even for a few minutes a day, you're likely to feel less stressed.

- Use your energy to focus on wellness and what you can do to stay as healthy as possible.

- Think about ways you can relax, such as relaxation exercises, yoga, or short meditations, and remove unneeded stressors from your life, if you can.

- Exercise and be as active as you can; it will help you to feel more fit and can lift your spirits. And, as we'll learn later in this chapter, some studies are now suggesting that regular exercise can reduce the risk of recurrences for some cancer survivors.

- Don't be afraid to seek professional counseling if your worries start to interfere with your life.

health for cancer survivors, look for the National Cancer Institute booklet, *Facing Forward: Life After Cancer Treatment*, at www.cancer.gov.) It includes a plan for treatment of any aftereffects of cancer or the therapies you received and a strategy for dealing with any ongoing health-maintenance issues, medical tests, or medications. You'll definitely want

What Should You Look For If You Are Concerned About Recurrence?

- Return of the cancer symptoms you had before
- New or unusual pain that's not related to an injury and doesn't go away
- Weight loss without trying
- Bleeding or unexplained bruising
- A rash or allergic reaction such as swelling, severe itching, or wheezing
- Chills or fevers that persist
- Headaches that don't go away
- Shortness of breath
- Bloody stools or blood in your urine
- Lumps, bumps, or swellings
- Nausea, vomiting, diarrhea, loss of appetite, or trouble swallowing
- A cough that doesn't go away
- Any other signs or symptoms mentioned by your doctor or nurse that you can't explain[3]

Many of these symptoms also can be signs of other illnesses or problems and may not mean that your cancer has returned. However, you should discuss them with your healthcare provider.[3]

to discuss when and what kind of tests you'll need as follow-up cancer screenings. The type and timing of screenings will vary depending on the type of cancer you had, your overall health, and other factors. Make sure that your oncologist and your primary-care doctor are in regular communication.

It's also good to talk with your healthcare provider about any concerns you have about the possible effects of cancer on your partner relationship, sexual functioning, work, and parenting. You also can ask for a referral to a counselor if you feel you need this support.

Your healthcare provider may have some specific recommendations for you to safeguard your health. These measures may include diet, exercise, getting to a healthy weight, using sunscreen, and stopping smoking. You also may want to consider whether or not you will curtail your intake of alcohol. Although consuming modest amounts of alcohol has healthy effects on the heart, it may increase the risk for some cancers.

If you are concerned about your family's risk of cancer—for instance, that your children may be at increased risk because of your cancer—you also might discuss recommendations for these family members with your clinician. You also can ask what the signs of recurrence are for your type of cancer and what symptoms should prompt you to see your oncologist or healthcare provider.

Once treatment is over, you also should have a written summary of the therapies you received from your oncologist. This written summary will describe any follow-up care that's needed. And these recommendations can be shared with any new doctors you see, as well as your primary-care doctor.

Health records you should keep include[4]

- The date your cancer was diagnosed
- The type of cancer for which you were treated
- Pathology reports on your cancer
- Details of operations, radiation treatment, and chemotherapy, including the names of drugs and dosages
- Any ongoing treatments to prevent the cancer from recurring, such as tamoxifen for breast cancer
- Key lab reports, X-rays, computed tomographic (CT) scans, and magnetic resonance imaging (MRI) studies
- A written list of signs and symptoms for which you should watch out
- Contact information for all the healthcare professionals involved in your treatment and follow-up care

It should be emphasized that it's very important to keep screening appointments after your treatment ends. These screenings can help to catch any cancer early, when it is more treatable. You also should be sure to take any medication that's prescribed, particularly if the medication will reduce the risk of your cancer recurring.

Unfortunately, for many reasons, cancer survivors don't always take their medications. For instance, breast cancer survivors often don't take the hormonal therapy drugs, such as tamoxifen and aromatase inhibitors, that are prescribed that can help to keep their cancer from recurring owing to uncomfortable side effects. One recent summary of studies found that 23% to 28% of women prescibed tamoxifen or aromatase inhibitors while enrolled in clinical trials discontinued their oral therapies earlier than recommended.[7] Women who've had breast cancers that are *hormone-sensitive*—that is, they're sensitive to the amount of hormones in their bodies—may be prescribed these drugs to reduce their risk of recurrence. The problem is that these drugs have bothersome side effects—including hot flashes, vaginal dryness, and nausea from tamoxifen and joint pain from aromatase inhibitors.

Yet it's vital that you keep taking any medication prescribed during and after cancer treatment for preventing recurrences. It's also important to continue to take prescribed medications if you are still "living with cancer." It's your best bet for reducing the risk of the disease or for battling it. And if side effects trouble you, talk with your physician. You often can switch to another drug or another type of drug that may help to reduce your risk but with fewer side effects.

"One of the first and foremost things to reduce the risk of recurrence for breast cancer survivors is to be adherent with treatment," says Susan Brown, manager of health education for Susan G. Komen for the Cure. "Unfortunately, some studies show that adherence with medications is not very good among breast cancer survivors long term. With the passage of time, women may forget the importance of their medication, and the burden of side effects becomes more problematic."

Brown notes that if the side effects of your medication trouble you, it's time to have a discussion with your healthcare provider about what you can do to ease these problems. Often there are medications or home remedies that can ease unwanted side effects such as hot flashes. Or another medication that can reduce your risk of cancer recurrence may be a good choice for you. It's also vital to keep your follow-up appointments with your oncologist, to see your primary healthcare clinician regularly, and to talk with your doctor about any health problems that persist after treatment.

Although many survivors return to normal function and activity level after treatment, others may suffer some health effects afterward. These can include neuropathy or problems with nerve function (often signaled by weakness or numbness in the hands or feet), pain, fatigue, cognitive or sexual difficulties, and elevated levels of anxiety or depression.[8] Some of these problems have to do with having had cancer; others are side effects of treatment. Some treatments, such as certain chemotherapies, also raise the risk of conditions such as osteoporosis and heart disease, so survivors need to be monitored by their physicians for these conditions after treatment.

"Cancer survivors are at risk for a number of conditions after treatment," says Kevin Stein, PhD, director for quality of life research for the Behavioral Research Center of the American Cancer Society. "So it's important for survivors to have regular medical care, as well as to discuss their health risks with their clinicians. Regular surveillance by a trusted healthcare team who can keep a keen eye out for troubling symptoms is one way to prevent and manage any aftereffects of cancer and its treatment."

Reducing the Risk of Cancer Recurrence

Many survivors have questions about other ways they can reduce their risk of recurrence. Often these questions have to do with vitamins and other dietary supplements. However, the most powerful lifestyle changes you can make to reduce risk are actually the most obvious—stop smoking, use sunscreen, protect yourself from infection (for more on this issue, see Chapter 7), maintain or attain a healthy weight, be physically active (within the constraints of any disabilities or limitations you may have), and choose a healthful diet with plenty of vegetables and fruits.[9]

Healthy weight is quite important for cancer survivors, according to the American Cancer Society's guidelines for nutrition and physical activity during and after cancer treatment.[9] Being too thin as well as being overweight or obese is a concern for cancer survivors. Some cancers and cancer treatments can lead to changes in eating patterns (because of side effects such as nausea, changes to taste, and mouth irritation) that make people lose weight and can even lead to malnutrition. Overweight patients, however, have a higher risk of recurrence for cancers such as those of the breast and prostate. They also have a higher risk for other health problems, such as high cholesterol, high blood pressure, diabetes, and heart disease.[9]

For cancer survivors who have a reduced appetite, eating smaller, more frequent meals without liquids can increase food intake. Fortified and commercially prepared nutrient-dense beverages or foods can improve calorie intake. For those who are overweight, losing weight— even a small amount—is beneficial. Weight loss of even 5% to 10% is thought to have significant health benefits.[9]

For their diet, survivors should strive for good nutrition—good nutrition not only may help to reduce cancer risk but can decrease your chance of conditions such as heart disease and diabetes and contribute to overall health, according to the American Cancer Society guidelines. It's wise to balance fat, protein, and carbohydrate. Eating lots of fruits and vegetables is key to maintaining a healthy weight. Although studies on cancer survivors do not agree on whether diets high in fruits and vegetables affect recurrences, some studies have suggested that such diets may affect the risk of recurrence of some cancers (such as those of the breast, prostate, and ovaries).[9] Eating whole grains is also important. Some studies have found that whole grains reduce the risk of initially developing cancer, although most of these studies have not looked at survivors' risk of recurrence. Still, whole grains add important nutrition and are a source of fiber in the diet as well.

The Question of Dietary Supplements

After cancer treatment, many survivors take dietary supplements in the hope that they can reduce the risk of cancer recurrence. However, there's very little support for the idea that supplements reduce cancer risk, and there's evidence of harm from some supplements, particularly in cancer survivors. Some supplements also can interfere with the effectiveness of cancer treatment. For instance, a study in 2004 in the *Journal of Clinical Oncology* found that nine popular herbal supplements, including echinacea, soy supplements, St. John's wort, ginseng, and kava, may interfere or interact with certain medications for cancer.[10,11]

What you hear or read about concerning dietary supplements is often based on anecdotal evidence—that is, someone's personal experience rather than scientific studies. Be skeptical of sources that make claims about supplements based on a few people's testimonials or vague references to scientific proof. Like drugs, dietary supplements can have risks and side effects. Unlike prescription drugs, though, claims about effectiveness of dietary supplements are not reviewed by the US Food and Drug Administration (FDA). So claims about a supplement you see on the Internet—such as those that claim to enhance immune function, for instance— may be entirely unsubstantiated by scientific evidence.[12]

If you are a cancer survivor, there may be some benefit in taking a multiple vitamin and mineral supplement that contains 100% of the recommended daily values, particularly if you feel you are not getting enough nutrients through your diet.[9] But large-dose vitamins, minerals, or other dietary supplements actually may be unhealthy and *increase your risk* for cancer and other health problems. (For more information on dietary supplements, see Chapter 4.)

Sticking to a low-fat diet is also a good practice for cancer survivors. Adequate low-fat protein intake (from fish and poultry and, to a lesser extent, lean meat) is crucial. Fat should comprise no more than 20% to 35% of calories. Whether low-fat diets influence the recurrence of cancer is open to question, although some studies have linked *saturated fat* with increasing cancer risk. However, we do know that low-fat diets such as those low in saturated fats and *trans* fats decrease the chance of heart disease, and high-fat diets increase the risk of obesity, which, in turn, increases the risk of cancer and cancer recurrence. Foods that are rich in omega-3 fatty acids (found in foods such as fish and walnuts) are also associated with a lower risk for heart disease.[9]

If you're a cancer survivor, you might want to limit alcohol. Studies have found a link between alcohol intake, especially high alcohol intake, and various types of cancer. Alcohol intake could affect the risk of new cancers, particularly of the mouth, throat, larynx, esophagus, liver, breast, and colon.[9]

The American Cancer Society guidelines also recommend limiting the intake of red and processed meats to decrease the risk of colorectal, prostate, and stomach cancers. No studies have looked at the influence of red or processed meats on cancer progression or recurrence, but it's probably wise to limit your intake of these meats, especially those cooked at high temperatures. It's thought that frying, broiling, or grilling red meats at very high temperatures increases the risk of some types of cancer.[9]

Cancer Survival: A Time to Get Moving?

As a cancer survivor, there are several important reasons for you to exercise. Regular exercise helps you to lose weight or maintain a healthy weight. It also may help to ease some of the physical problems that can trouble you after treatment, such as muscle loss and fatigue. Exercise is also helpful for reducing the risk of conditions that sometimes can occur after cancer treatment, such as osteoporosis and heart disease. And a few studies even suggest that exercise can reduce the risk of cancer recurrence, especially for breast and colon cancer survivors.[9]

At the same time, beginning an exercise program—a challenging task even for those who are healthy—can be difficult for cancer survivors because of the physical problems they may experience after treatment. If you find exercise taxing after treatment, however, it's important to know that even a little bit of exercise can be beneficial. And exercise need not be very strenuous to improve your health.

As we noted in Chapter 5, several new and exciting studies have reported the benefits of exercise for cancer survivors. In two studies, women with a history of breast cancer who exercised for more than 2 to 3 hours per week had a significantly lower risk of death or breast cancer recurrence compared with women who were sedentary. Although the studies showed that physical activity was beneficial for all women after a diagnosis of breast cancer, those who were diagnosed with higher stages of the disease and who had estrogen receptor–positive tumors got the most benefit in terms of avoiding breast cancer recurrence.

There are several reasons why exercise may reduce the risk of breast cancer recurrence: Exercise helps to reduce weight and body fat, thus lowering circulating levels of hormones that can feed breast cancer growth. Physical activity also improves insulin resistance and reduces the risk of diabetes, which has been tied to the risk of a number of cancers, including breast, colon, pancreas, and endometrial cancers.[14]

Two other studies published in 2006 also found that physical activity can improve survival and reduce cancer recurrence significantly in people with nonmetastatic colon cancer (cancer that has not spread to distant parts of the body).[15,16] When combined with standard therapies, higher levels of physical activity contributed to a 50% reduced risk of recurrence and mortality. These studies provide preliminary evidence that exercise reduces the risk of recurrence for cancer survivors, and other new research is continuing to delve into this subject.

How much exercise and what kind are the best for cancer survivors? These are very individual questions and will depend on your age, overall health and fitness, and previous activity level, as well as your personal risk factors for cancer and other conditions. The jury is still out on how much exercise it takes to reduce the risk of breast or colorectal cancer recurrence, but studies that showed a reduction in risk found the most benefit for those who were physically active for at least 2 to 3 hours per week, according to a review of studies on cancer risk and physical activity published in *Nature Reviews Cancer* in 2008.[14]

Resistance exercise, as well as aerobic exercise, is also good for building up any muscle lost during treatment and for reducing the risk of the bone-thinning disease *osteoporosis*, which troubles many people after menopause and in their older years. Because young women who undergo cancer treatment sometimes experience menopause during or after treatment, and because men with prostate cancer are treated long term with hormone-suppressing medications, they are at increased risk for osteoporosis. The reason is that our body's hormones help to build bone. Resistance training also has the additional benefit of improving lean body mass and balance, which reduces the risk of falls and fractures.

Cancer survivors with lymphedema may benefit from range-of-motion exercises to improve this condition—with approval from their treating physician, according to the American Cancer Society's guidelines for nutrition and physical activity during and after cancer treatment. Strength training was once suspected of exacerbating lymphedema, but recent research indicates that slowly progressive weight lifting is safe and actually appears to improve lymphedema and reduce symptoms. Survivors should check with their physician before embarking on any physical activity program. Because survivors with neuropathy may have a reduced ability to use their affected limbs owing to weakness or loss of balance, their choice of exercise should take these problems into consideration. For instance, they may do better using a reclining stationary bicycle than exercising on a treadmill.[9] Studies do show that exercise in cancer survivors can improve mood, reduce anxiety and depression, increase self-esteem, and decrease symptoms of fatigue. So there are many reasons to be active. However, if you feel that you'll have trouble starting or maintaining an exercise program on your own, it may be a good time to seek help from a physical therapist or exercise specialist. Survivors should seek exercise training from those who are certified by an exercise-related professional organization, such as the American College of Sports Medicine.[9]

How do you start an exercise program? If you are sedentary, any choices you can make that can move you toward an active lifestyle are wise ones. Start out with short walks or 10-minute stretching sessions, and gradually build up your exercise sessions when you have more stamina. If you are exercising three times a week, try to increase these sessions to five times a week. Keep in mind, though, that moderate exercise should be your mantra—you don't have to walk a marathon!

There are some cautions for cancer survivors when embarking on exercise, especially if you are still undergoing treatment. In addition to discussing your exercise plans with your doctor, taking the following precautions is a good idea, according to the American Cancer Society guidelines.[9]

- If you have severe anemia, delay exercise until the anemia has improved.
- If you have compromised immune function, avoid public gyms until your white cell blood count returns to normal. Those who have received a bone marrow transplant should avoid going to public gyms for 1 year after treatment.
- Those suffering from severe fatigue should try just 10 minutes of stretching daily.
- Survivors with indwelling catheters should avoid water or other conditions that might increase the risk of infections, as

well as resistance training because this type of exercise can dislodge catheters.

- If you have received cardiotoxic therapies, talk with your doctor about if, how much, and what kind of exercise may be right for you.

Heart Disease, Diabetes, and Osteoporosis

It's been said that the experience of cancer changes one's life forever. In addition to experiencing a range of emotions after a cancer diagnosis, such as fear, depression, and anxiety, you're likely to experience physical changes that may persist after treatment is finished.

Also, cancer survivors are at increased risk for other major health conditions, such as heart disease, osteoporosis, and diabetes, because of their cancer and some treatments. The symptoms you may have will depend on the type of cancer you had and its treatment. Let's talk about risk for heart disease, diabetes, and osteoporosis—because they can easily threaten the health of cancer survivors—and how you can reduce your risk.

Heart Disease

The chemotherapy, radiation, or other treatment that you may have received for cancer also can have a serious side effect—an increased risk for heart disease. It's rare to have heart disease from a treatment soon after cancer treatment, but cancer survivors—particularly long-term cancer survivors who received treatment as children—are at risk for the development of heart disease months or years later. The reason is that some chemotherapies and other therapies, such as radiation to the chest area, can damage the muscle cells in the heart, resulting in changes in blood pressure, heart arrhythmias, and in rare cases congestive heart failure. Today, drugs you receive during treatment can lessen the chance of cardiac toxicity. Technical improvements in administering chemotherapy and radiation therapy and in detecting early signs of heart problems also have made such side effects less likely.[17,18]

However, cancer survivors do have more risk of having heart problems when compared with the rest of the population. These conditions can be especially problematic for people who had heart disease before they started treatment or are elderly. Most often, however, they can be managed with cardiovascular disease medications.

What Can You Do to Be as Heart Healthy as Possible if You Are a Survivor?

The most important step is to have regular cardiac evaluations by your doctor. Depending on your medical history, this may mean a regular physical examination and management of conditions such as high blood pressure with medicines. It even may include an echocardiogram, or a scan of the heart, if your healthcare provider feels that you are at risk. Report any symptoms of heart disease, such as breathlessness and change in your pulse or heartbeat, to your doctor right away. Other ways you can prevent cardiovascular disease include exercising, stopping smoking, and eating a diet low in fats, particularly saturated and *trans* fat.[17,18]

Osteoporosis

Some survivors, particularly those treated for breast and prostate cancer, are at risk for osteoporosis. Osteoporosis is a condition in which the bones become less dense and more likely to fracture. Osteoporosis is often called a "silent" disease because it can progress undetected for many years and is sometimes diagnosed only after a fracture occurs.

People treated for breast and prostate cancer are at risk for osteoporosis because chemotherapy, surgery, or medications that decrease the risk of recurrence also can reduce levels of circulating hormones throughout the body. These hormones help to build bone, so their loss can trigger osteoporosis. Some young women undergoing breast cancer chemotherapy also can go through early menopause, which also brings with it loss of circulating hormones. So even young women who've had breast cancer can be at risk for osteoporosis. If you are at risk for osteoporosis, you should be sure to get regular bone density scans. These tests can detect osteoporosis before a fracture occurs and predict one's risk for fracture in the future. Although there are effective medications for osteoporosis, the best way to stop this condition is to prevent it. According to the National Institutes of Health Osteoporosis and Related Bone Diseases National Resource Center, some strategies for preventing osteoporosis include[19]

- *Eating a diet high in calcium and vitamin D.* Good sources of calcium include low-fat dairy products, dark-green leafy vegetables, and calcium-fortified foods. Foods with vitamin D include fortified cereals and milk. A calcium supplement with vitamin D also may be a good idea. According to the Institute of Medicine of the National Academies, those younger than age 50 should have an intake of at least 1000 mg of calcium a day, and those older than age 50 should strive to increase their intake to 1200 mg. The recommended intake for vitamin D is 200 International Units (IU) for those aged 50 years and younger, 400 IU for those aged 51 to 70 years, and 600 IU for those 71 years of age and older.

- *Doing weight-bearing exercise that can help strengthen your bones.* This kind of exercise forces you to work against gravity. Weight-bearing exercise includes walking, climbing stairs, lifting weight, and dancing.
- *Stopping smoking and reducing alcohol consumption if you drink heavily.* Smoking is bad for the bones and causes you to absorb less calcium from your diet. Some studies also indicate that drinking too much alcohol may negatively affect bone health.

Diabetes

Some medicines for breast and prostate cancer also can increase the risk for diabetes. And diabetes is a health threat even if you haven't had cancer. More than 23 million people in the United States have diabetes, and unfortunately, almost 6 million are unaware that they have the disease, according to the American Diabetes Association. Prediabetes is also a serious medical condition. This is a problem in which blood sugars become elevated, and it can lead to type 2 diabetes if left unchecked.

The good news is that even those with prediabetes can prevent the development of type 2 diabetes with a combination of healthy diet and physical activity. The recent Diabetes Prevention Program study, for instance, showed that people with prediabetes can prevent type 2 diabetes with these measures and even return their blood glucose level to a normal healthy range. According to the American Diabetes Association, steps to prevent diabetes include[20]

- Eat a variety of foods, including vegetables, whole grains, fruits, nonfat dairy products, beans, and lean meats, poulty and fish.
- Watch your portion sizes.
- Pick foods that are rich in vitamins, minerals, and fiber over those that are processed.
- Aim for at least 30 minutes of physical activity each day. Good physical activities include walking, gardening, swimming, or even

cleaning house. For the most benefit, physical activity should raise your heart rate and cause you to break into a light sweat.

- For the most benefit from exercise, include activities that are aerobic, provide strength training, and keep you flexible. Aerobic exercise increases your heart rate, works your muscles, and raises your breathing rate. These exercises include activities such as walking, dancing, and swimming. Strength training means building strong bones and muscles by working with weights, elastic bands, or plastic tubes. Flexibility exercises are those that gently stretch your muscles, keeping your joints flexible and reducing the risk of injury from physical activity.

Resources for Cancer Survivors

National Cancer Institute. *Facing Forward: Life after Cancer Treatment.* Available at www.cancer.gov/cancertopics/life-after-treatment/.

American Cancer Society. *Information for Survivors.* Available at www.cancer.org/docroot/HOME/srv/srv_0.asp.

American Cancer Society Cancer Survivors Network: www.acscsn.org/index.html?popup=1.

Cure Magazine—for cancer survivors. Available at www.curetoday.com/.

Mamm magazine—for breast and reproductive cancer survivors, Available at www.mamm.com/.

Women & Cancer Magazine—for women concerned about cancer prevention and surviviorship. Available at www.awomanshealth.com

References

1. American Cancer Society. *Cancer Facts and Figures 2009.* Available at www.cancer.org/docroot/STT/content/STT_1x_Cancer_Facts__Figures_2009.asp?from=fast. Accessed January 21, 2010.

2. National Cancer Institute. *New Malignancies Among Cancer Survivors: SEER Cancer Registries, 1973–2000.* Available at http://seer.cancer.gov/publications/mpmono/.

3. American Cancer Society. *Living with Uncertainty: The Fear of Cancer Recurrence.* Available at www.cancer.org/docroot/MLT/content/MLT_4_1x_Living_With_Uncertainty_-_The_Fear_of_Cancer_Recurrence.asp. Accessed August 10, 2009.

4. National Cancer Institute. *Facing Forward: Life after Cancer Treatment.* Available at www.cancer.gov/cancertopics/life-after-treatment/. Accessed October 18, 2008.

5. Institute of Medicine. *From Cancer Patient to Cancer Survivor: Lost in Transition. Report Recommendations. Fact Sheet,* November 2005. Available at www.iom.edu/CMS/28312/4931/30869/34764.aspx. Accessed August 8, 2009.

6. Institute of Medicine. *From Cancer Patient to Cancer Survivor. Lost in Transition. Cancer Survivorship Care Planning. Fact Sheet,* November 2005. Available at www.iom.edu/CMS/28312/4931/30869/30879.aspx. Accessed August 8, 2009

7. Ruddy K, Mayer E, Partridge A. Patient adherence and persistence with oral anticancer treatment. *CA Cancer J Clin.* 2009;59:56–66.

8. Stein KD, Syrjala KL, Andrykowski MA. Physical and psychological long-term and late effects of cancer. *Cancer.* 2008;112:S2577-S2592.

9. Doyle C, Kushi LH, Byers T, et al. Nutrition and physical activity during and after cancer treatment: an American Cancer Society Guide for Informed Choices. *CA Cancer J Clin.* 2006;56:323–353.

10. Sparreboom A, Cox MC, Acharya MR, Figg WD. Herbal remedies in the United States: potential adverse interactions with anticancer agents. *J Clin Oncol.* 2004;22:2489–2503.

11. Brower V. An apple a day may be safer than vitamins. *J Natl Cancer Inst.* 2008;100:770–772.

12. American Cancer Society. *Dietary Supplements: How to Know What Is Safe.* Available at www.cancer.org/docroot/ETO/content/ETO_5_3x_How_to_Know_What_Is_Safe_Choosing_and_Using_Dietary_Supplements.asp. Accessed January 21, 2010.

13. American Cancer Society. *Nutrition and Physical Activity during and after Cancer Treatment: Answers to Common Questions.* Available at www.cancer.org/docroot/mbc/content/MBC_6_2x_FAQ_Nutrition_and_Physical_Activity.asp. Accessed October 18, 2008.

14. McTiernan A. Mechanisms linking physical activity with cancer. *Nat Rev Cancer.* 2008;8:205–211.

15. Meyerhardt JA, Giovannucci El, Holmes MD, et al. Physical activity and survival after colorectal cancer diagnosis. *J Clin Oncol.* 2006;24:3527–3234.

16. Meryerhardt JA, Hesletine D, Niedzwiecki D, et al. Impact of physical activity on cancer recurrence and survival in patients with stage III colon cancer: findings from CALGB 89803. *J Clin Oncol.* 2006;24:3535–3541.

17. Whitttington E. Keeping heart-healthy during and after cancer treatment. *CureExtra.* Summer 2005.

18. Stakeholders report: the cancer survivors prescription for living. *Am J Nurs.* April 2007. Available at www.nursingcenter.com/library/static.asp?pageid=701558. Accessed August 9, 2009

19. National Institutes of Health, Osteoporosis and Related Bone Diseases Resource Center. *What Breast Cancer Survivors Need to Know about Osteoporosis Fact Sheet*, Available at http://www.niams.nih.gov/Health_Info/Bone/Osteoporosis/Conditions_Behaviors/osteoporosis_breast_cancer.asp. Accessed January 21, 2010.

20. American Diabetes Association. *How to Prevent or Delay Diabetes*. Available at www.diabetes.org/food-nutrition-lifestyle/lifestyle-prevention/prevention/how-to-prevent-or-delay-diabetes.jsp. Accessed August 27, 2009.

12

Stress Busters: Staying Positive
One Day at a Time

The idea that stress is associated with cancer is a common one.[1] If only we could reduce the stress in our lives, then we could prevent cancer or recover from it more easily, according to some.

Is this true? For decades, modern scientific investigators have tested the relationship between stress and cancer, and the results so far have been glaringly inconclusive. In fact, there's little hard scientific evidence that stressful life events or even the amount of self-perceived stress in one's life significantly affects cancer risk.[1-4]

However, stress is interwoven with cancer risk in other ways. There's no doubt that being at increased risk for cancer—or going through the diagnosis and treatment of cancer—is stressful.

So, for those who are at risk, and for cancer survivors, this chapter is meant to be a guide to stress-reduction techniques, including methods ranging from meditation to yoga. We'll discuss what the research says about these approaches and then provide some tips for practicing them. But first let's consider the question of whether stress leads to cancer because it's an important one.

Studies done over the past 30 years have looked at whether stress causes cancer, but they have produced conflicting results. Although some studies have indicated a link between stress and cancer risk, a direct cause-and-effect relationship hasn't been proven, according to the National Cancer Institute. What are the reasons for these inconsistent study results? It's often difficult to separate stress from other physical and emotional factors when examining cancer risk. For example, researchers may have difficulty separating the effects of stress from behaviors or life-style factors such as smoking, using alcohol and becoming overweight or biological factors such as becoming older or having a family history of cancer. All these factors can have an impact on cancer risk.[5]

Several recent reviews of scientific evidence by Danish, French, and Dutch researchers have found that although there's been a vast amount of research into the question of stress and cancer, a conclusive link hasn't been proven. However, a review of 70 studies published in 2004 found that there was some evidence that experiencing losses or having a low level of social support contributed to an unfavorable prognosis in those with cancer. Still, the researchers concluded that the evidence of an association was rather weak.[2-4] One large study published in 2006 in the *British Journal of Cancer*, in which more than 10,000 people were surveyed and then followed for up to 11 years, did not find that self-reported stressful life events affected or increased cancer risk. However, those who reported more stressful life events also said that they had poorer health behaviors, including alcohol and tobacco consumption (which can affect cancer risk).[1] According to the American Cancer Society, some research has shown that major life stressors such as divorce or the death of a loved one can raise cancer risk slightly. Poverty is linked to higher cancer risk, but this may be more related to poor access to medical care than to the stress of poverty itself. Yet it's interesting to note that studies have shown that people who are more socially isolated are more likely to die of all causes, including cancer.[6]

How does stress affect people who already have cancer? According to the National Cancer Institute, stress *may* affect tumor growth and spread and *may* weaken the immune system.[5] But, again, the relationship has not been consistently linked in studies. At the same time, it's difficult to know how to interpret the results of these studies because cancer is a stressful experience—so does the stress come before the cancer has spread or because of it?

A subject that's closely related to the issue of stress and cancer risk is the question of whether certain personality traits or psychological factors can affect cancer incidence. These traits or psychological factors include depression, anxiety, the tendency to feel helpless, and the tendency to suppress negative emotions. Researchers, as well as the public, have long been interested in whether such psychological factors can influence cancer risk.

Like research concerning stress and cancer, however, studies on whether psychological factors affect cancer risk have been somewhat contradictory. Recent reviews or summaries of scientific studies, however, have found that the total evidence for a link between psychological factors and cancer risk is weak or inconclusive.[3,4,7]

Several large studies on psychological factors and cancer risk also have failed to find an association. In one study published in the *Journal of the National Cancer Institute* in 2008, researchers followed over 9000 Dutch women who had completed a personality questionnaire. Those who developed breast cancer over 13 years were compared with those who did not. The researchers considered whether a variety of personality traits or psychological coping styles were more common in the women with breast cancer. These included a tendency to repress emotions and to control anger as well as traits such as exhibiting nonassertiveness, depression, and an attitude of helplessness or hopelessness. The scientists' conclusion was that none of these psychological factors was associated with the development of breast cancer.[8]

Likewise, a study of more than 1000 patients with head and neck cancer failed to find a link between emotional well-being and survival. Over time, those who scored highest on tests of emotional well-being showed no differences in cancer growth or the length of time they survived compared with those with lower scores. [9]

Either way, it's important to know that we have a long way to go in researching the interrelationships among cancer, stress, and psychology. If stress or psychological factors play any role in cancer development, it is probably just one small piece of the pie. It's also vital to realize that the belief that psychological stress or certain personality traits lead to cancer can lead to a dangerous tendency to "blame the victim." It can lead to the type of thinking that says, "Well, if you didn't have a certain personality type or you were more positive, then you wouldn't have cancer!" And this is a belief that can make any cancer survivor feel disheartened. It's more helpful to focus on the ways stress reduction can benefit those at risk for cancer and those who have experienced the disease. One large study published in 2007, for instance, found that having a personal or family history of cancer significantly increased psychological distress, as well as levels of anxiety and depression.[10] This study illustrates the need for stress reduction among those who are at risk and who are cancer survivors. And studies have well documented the benefits of stress reduction: Stress-reduction methods such as meditation improve positive mood, decrease insomnia, relieve anxiety , and even help to alleviate chronic pain.[11]

To talk about stress reduction, we first have to consider what stress means. *Stress* is the way the body defends itself when it's challenged. In response to a certain event—whether it's outright physical danger, a tough life situation, or even making a presentation at work—your body activates your nervous system and certain hormones. Your body produces the hormones epinephrine (adrenaline) and cortisol—speeding up breathing, heart rate, and blood pressure. Your entire body goes on alert as blood flows to your muscles, your pupils dilate to enhance vision, and you produce sweat to cool your skin. All these reactions are the body's way of dealing with pressure and sometimes danger. When working properly, the stress response helps you to perform at your best. However, when stress goes into overdrive—when it is chronic or an exaggerated response to the situation at hand—it can cause physical symptoms and even may contribute to health conditions, such as insomnia, chronic headaches, reduction in one's tolerance for pain, anxiety, depression, and even high blood pressure.[12]

Tips From the Experts: Stress Relievers

There are a number of techniques and therapies that seem to help people reduce stressful feelings, ranging from exercise to meditation. We'll talk about each of these techniques in turn, but first, here are a few general tips on managing stress in your life from the American Academy of Family Physicians and the National Women's Health Information Center[13,16]:

- *Try to find time to relax*, even if it's just a few minutes per day.
- *Make time for yourself.* No matter how busy you are, you can set aside at least 15 minutes a day to do something nice for yourself, such as going for a walk or calling a friend.
- *Set realistic goals for yourself at home and at work.* No one expects you to be perfect. If you need help—especially if you're dealing with cancer—ask for support from friends or family, or seek out a counselor. Talking about the stress you feel can help. Work to resolve conflicts with other people.
- *Eat nutritious meals and get enough sleep.*
- *Compromise.* Sometimes it's not worth the stress to argue.
- *Set limits.* When it comes to things such as work and family, figure out what you can realistically do. Don't be afraid to say no to requests for your time and energy.
- *Make time for yourself to exercise and to explore hobbies that interest you.*

Dealing with the aftereffects of cancer, even after treatment is finished, can be stressful. Some physical changes you may experience can bring on troubling emotions as well—making you feel nervous, anxious, or even depressed. We asked Kevin Stein, PhD, director of quality of life research for the Behavioral Research Center of the American Cancer Society, for some tips on coping with these emotions. Here are some suggestions:

- Exercise can help you to feel better physically as well as emotionally.

- Know that you may feel anxious or depressed at certain times after your treatment is finished—such as on the anniversary of your diagnosis or when you are scheduled for follow-up tests.

- Try some stress-management techniques to control anxiety:
  - Practice deep breathing.
  - Use guided imagery. Picture yourself on a pleasant beach or in the forest to lower your anxiety or stress level.
  - Use progressive relaxation. Lie down in a quiet place, and imagine each muscle group from head to toe gradually relaxing deeper and deeper.
  - Use cognitive reframing. If you have a negative or stressful thought, replace it with a positive one, such as, "I can make it through this experience."

If your stress, anxiety, or depression starts interfering with your daily functioning or is persistent, it may be time to seek professional help. Psychological counseling and antidepressant or antianxiety medication or both can be helpful in these cases.

If a stressful situation is long term, it can produce chronic low-level anxiety that's difficult for many people to tolerate. It can make you feel fatigued or overwhelmed or depressed or anxious and even can weaken your immune system. What are the signs of stress? They include the following[13]:

- Anxiety
- Chronic back pain

- Constipation or diarrhea
- Depression
- Difficulty concentrating or making decisions
- Fatigue
- Headaches
- High blood pressure
- Insomnia
- Mood swings
- Nightmares
- Problems with relationships
- Shortness of breath
- Stiff neck
- Upset stomach
- Unintentional weight gain or loss

If you have any of these symptoms, it's possible that there may be reasons for them other than stress. So having one of these symptoms may mean that you should consult with your doctor to see if there is a medical reason for them. Yet, even if these symptoms are caused by a medical condition, it's possible that stress can make them worse.

If you are a cancer survivor or someone who is at increased risk for cancer, some signs that you may need to learn to manage stress include[14]

- Thinking about cancer the first thing in the morning and the last thing every night
- Being so worried about cancer that it affects your relationships and enjoyment of activities
- Being upset even by minor aches and pains
- Feeling overwhelmed and unable to manage your life
- Thinking that your friends or family don't understand you

According to the National Comprehensive Cancer Network, cancer-related distress can include everything from normal feelings of vulnerability, sadness, and fear to problems that can become disabling, such as depression, anxiety, panic, and social isolation. If you feel that you have serious distress about having cancer that is interfering with your daily activities, it's important to seek help in the form of counseling from a mental health professional or pastoral caregiver experienced in treating those with cancer. Taking care of yourself if you experience cancer-related distress is vital for your well-being as well as your quality of life.[15]

There are also some other regular practices and approaches to reducing stress that may work for you. These include aerobic exercise, such as walking, as well as relaxing types of exercise, such as yoga, stretching, and tai chi. Studies show that mind/body therapies such as meditation also may decrease stress. Following is some information about a few of these stress-reduction methods and tips on getting the most out of each type of therapy or practice.

Exercise: Why It Reduces Stress*

Exercise may improve mental health by helping the brain cope better with stress, according to research into the effect of exercise on neurochemicals involved in the body's stress response. Preliminary evidence suggests that physically active people have lower rates of anxiety and depression than sedentary people. But little work has focused on why that should be. So to determine how exercise might bring about its mental health benefits, some researchers are looking at possible links between exercise and brain chemicals associated with stress, anxiety, and depression.

So far there's little evidence for the popular theory that exercise causes a rush of endorphins. Rather, one line of research points to the less familiar neuromodulator norepinephrine, which may help the brain deal with stress more efficiently.

Work in animals since the late 1980s has found that exercise increases brain concentrations of norepinephrine in brain regions involved in the body's stress response.

Norepinephrine is particularly interesting to researchers because 50 percent of the brain's supply is produced in the locus coeruleus, a brain area that connects most of the brain regions involved in emotional and stress responses. The chemical is thought to play a major role in modulating the action of other, more prevalent neurotransmitters that play a direct role in the stress response. And although researchers are unsure of exactly how most antidepressants work, they know that some increase brain concentrations of norepinephrine.

But some psychologists don't think it's a simple matter of more norepinephrine equals less stress and anxiety and therefore less depression. Instead, they think exercise thwarts depression and anxiety by enhancing the body's ability to respond to stress.

Biologically, exercise seems to give the body a chance to practice dealing with stress. It forces the body's physiological systems—all of

*From the American Psychological Association's publication and fact sheet *Exercise Fuels the Brain's Stress Buffers*.[17] Thanks also to Rod K. Dishman, PhD, of the University of Georgia, and Mark Sothmann, PhD, of Indiana University's School of Medicine and School of Allied Health Sciences.

which are involved in the stress response—to communicate much more closely than usual: The cardiovascular system communicates with the renal system, which communicates with the muscular system. And all of these are controlled by the central and sympathetic nervous systems, which also must communicate with each other. This workout of the body's communication system may be the true value of exercise; the more sedentary we get, the less efficient are our bodies in responding to stress.

Yoga: Fitness the Relaxing Way

Yoga is everywhere today. Walk into any fitness center and you're likely to find a yoga class. In fact, an entire industry has grown up around this practice in the United States. You can easily find anything from yoga mats to yoga pants to home yoga CDs with any casual search on the Internet.

But yoga is more than a way to get fit and to relax. It's actually a discipline and philosophy that combines physical postures, breathing exercises, meditation, and behaviors aimed at achieving spiritual enlightenment. The term *yoga* actually comes from the Sanskrit work *yuj*, which means "yoke" or "union," and is believed to describe the union between mind and body. The first written text about yoga surfaced more than 2000 years ago in *The Yoga Sutras*, but yoga may have been practiced for as long as 5000 years. It was developed originally as a way for practitioners to achieve discipline and attain spiritual enlightenment. The eight spiritual "limbs," or foundations, of yoga include

- Yama (moral behavior)
- Niyama (healthy habits)
- Asana (physical postures)
- Pranayama (breathing exercises)
- Pratyahara (sense withdrawal)
- Dharana (concentration)
- Dhyana (contemplation)
- Samadhi (higher consciousness)

There are various schools of yoga, and all of them incorporate at least some of these limbs into their practice. Hatha yoga, which is the most common type in the United States, emphasizes postures (asanas) and breathing exercises (pranayama). Within hatha yoga, there are also various schools, ranging from Bikram to Iyengar to Kundalini. Some schools emphasize stretching, strength, and balance, whereas others use fluid movement from pose to pose to increase strength, flexibility, and fitness, also termed *power yoga*. A 2002 survey by the National Center for Health

Statistics and the National Center for Complementary and Alternative Medicine found that yoga is one of the top 10 "alternative" or "complementary" methods of medicine used in the United States. Nearly 8% of more than 31,000 participants in this survey had used yoga for health.

According to the National Center for Complementary and Alternative Medicine, research suggests that yoga might[18]

- Improve mood and a sense of well-being
- Reduce stress
- Decrease heart rate and blood pressure
- Increase lung capacity
- Improve muscle relaxation
- Relieve anxiety, depression, and insomnia
- Improve overall physical fitness, strength, and flexibility

I've used yoga as a way to relax and feel fit for years. Several times a week I roll out my yoga mat and put on a 20-minute CD that takes me through a variety of poses that stretch my body and demand muscle work. At the end of each session, I usually feel relaxed and strengthened—as if I've been through a good workout, but one that is easy for me to achieve. In fact, studies have found that yoga is safe in most healthy people and has few side effects. Most yoga classes today don't demand strenuous pretzel poses and are even safe (and beneficial) for those with limited motion, such as people with mild arthritis. Some poses require some muscle strength, a fair sense of balance, and the ability to sit straight and stretch. If you feel challenged by any particular pose, however, it's wise to sit it out and go on to poses you feel you can handle. However, there are some cautions from National Center for Complementary and Alternative Medicine regarding yoga[18].

- People with spinal disc disease, extremely high or low blood pressure, glaucoma, retinal detachment, fragile or atherosclerotic arteries, a risk of blood clots, ear problems, severe osteoporosis, or cervical spondylitis should avoid inverted poses.
- Pregnant women should consult with a yoga teacher about whether to avoid certain poses.
- If you have a medical condition, consult with your healthcare provider before beginning yoga.
- When you take yoga in a class, ask if the teacher is trained or certified.

Yoga is currently being studied for its effects on a range of health conditions, including depression, HIV infection, arthritis, insomnia, multiple sclerosis, and even smoking cessation! In the future, we may know more about the medical benefits of yoga, but for now, it seems to be a safe and fun way to practice stress reduction.

Tai Chi: Meditation in Motion

You've probably seen people practicing tai chi; the graceful dance-like poses of this art are a joy to watch.[19] However, tai chi—which originated in China as a martial art—also may have health benefits. For instance, one review study funded by the National Center for Complementary Medicine found that tai chi reduced participants' blood pressure in 22 of 26 studies. According to Chinese thought, tai chi helps the vital energy know as *qi* (pronounced "chee") to flow through the body, a process believed to bring health and well-being. Although these beliefs have not been proven by Western science, some studies suggest that tai chi does seem to have a few health benefits.

People who practice tai chi move their bodies in a slow, relaxed, and graceful series of movements, each flowing into the next. The body is in constant motion, and good posture is an important part of the practice, as is deep, relaxed, and focused breathing. You can practice on your own or in a group. Most practitioners of tai chi use deep breathing to concentrate on the movements and put distracting thoughts aside. These practices make tai chi a moving meditation that is thought to increase calmness and awareness, as well as overall health.

- Tai chi is considered to be a low-impact aerobic exercise, as well as a weight-bearing exercise, and thus it is suited for those who need to gently strengthen their bones or improve flexibility and strength. Some people use this art to help with coordination and balance and also to prevent falls, especially in the elderly. Some people also use tai chi for easing pain and stiffness from arthritis
- Improving sleep
- Decreasing anxiety, depression, and chronic pain
- Increasing fitness and muscle strength

However, it's important to keep in mind that tai chi is not a substitute for regular medical care. It may have some health benefits, but more research is needed to *prove* exactly how tai chi affects health. As with yoga, there are also important cautions for its use, including

- Consult with your healthcare provider if you have any chronic health condition and want to start tai chi.

- If you don't position your body properly or overdo practice, you can get sore muscles or sprains.
- Don't practice tai chi right after you eat, when you are very tired, or when you have an active infection.
- Consult with your healthcare provider about doing tai chi if you are pregnant or have a hernia, joint problems, back pain, sprains, a fracture, or severe osteoporosis.

Meditation: Mindful Relaxation

Meditation is a mind/body process that uses concentration or reflection to relax the body and calm the mind. Meditation is a commonly used approach to relieving stress, especially for cancer patients. Herbert Benson, MD, of the Benson-Henry Institute for Mind Body Medicine at Massachusetts General Hospital, has documented the effects of meditation on the body since the 1960s, and his research has shown that meditation[12]

- Decreases muscle tension
- Lowers blood pressure
- Eases anxiety and depression
- Relieves insomnia
- Helps patients to deal with chronic pain
- Also may relieve nausea associated with chemotherapy

Benson termed the state of deep relaxation achieved by meditation the "relaxation response." In meditation, the metabolism slows, the heart beats less rapidly, and blood is pumped through the arteries less forcefully, helping to lower blood pressure. The muscles relax, and the brain releases soothing hormones, such as serotonin. Says Dr. Benson, "It's like giving a hyperenergetic kindergartner an afternoon nap."[20]

Meditation is rooted in ancient Buddhism. It is based on the concept of being "mindful"—of focusing on the present rather than on the future or the past. Transcendental meditation originated in India and uses a word, sound, or phrase repeated silently to prevent distracting thoughts. The goal of any type of meditation is to settle both the mind and body into a quiet state and to achieve deep rest.[21]

Some cancer centers offer meditation and relaxation methods along with usual medical care. Although meditation can be helpful to cancer patients and survivors, it is not a substitute for conventional medical care. Nor does scientific evidence suggest that meditation can treat cancer or any other disease. What it can do, however, is improve quality of life for people with cancer and other chronic conditions.

There are several different types of meditation. In *concentrated meditation*, you focus on a sound, a mental picture, your breath, or a mantra—a meaningful word such as *peace* or one that has religious significance. By contrast, those who practice *awareness meditation* carefully notice and focus on their thoughts, feelings, and body sensations—even such small physical feelings as a twinge in the leg. In *expressive meditation*, you concentrate on a rhythmic activity such as jogging, dancing, or tai chi exercises.

Meditation can be self-directed or guided by doctors, psychiatrists, other mental health professionals, or masters from different schools of meditation. Meditation often involves choosing a quiet place free from distraction, sitting or resting quietly with the eyes closed, noticing breathing and physical sensations, and letting go of intruding thoughts.[11]

Learning meditation is not always easy, however. Many people often feel restless when they start learning to meditate and have trouble focusing their minds. For beginners, distracting thoughts often can interfere with meditation. However, over time, many people find that they can practice meditation more easily, and it seems to help them reduce the stress in their lives. One tip for beginners: If you find your attention wandering, just return your focus to the breath or mantra, but without judging yourself.

Whatever meditation technique you try, remember that it can be adapted to suit your needs. Some people may prefer a restful meditation versus an active one, whereas others may choose to focus on the spiritual aspects of meditation, repeating a word or phrase with personal significance to them. Others may find it easier and simpler just to relax and focus on the rhythm of their breathing. Following is a technique that Benson teaches to his patients. He recommends that it should be done for 10 to 20 minutes each day or twice daily.[12,20]

- Pick a focus word or short phrase that's rooted in your belief system, such as
  - *Peace* (secular)
  - *Om* (Hindu)
  - *Shalom* (Jewish)
  - *Insha'allah* (Islamic)
  - *Hail Mary, full of grace* (Catholic)
  - *The Lord is my shepherd* (Christian)
- Sit quietly in a comfortable position.
- Close your eyes and relax your muscles.
- Breathe slowly and naturally, and as you do, silently repeat your focus word, phrase, or prayer to yourself as you exhale.

- Assume a passive attitude. Don't worry about how well you're doing. When other thoughts come to mind, simply say to yourself, "Oh, well," and gently return to the repetition.

There's a lot of ongoing interesting research investigating the use of meditation and the ways it affects the body and mind. The National Center for Complementary and Alternative Medicine is currently funding clinical studies[21] that will study the effects of meditation on

- Preventing and treating heart disease
- Relieving symptoms of rheumatoid arthritis and lower back pain
- Emotional and cognitive (thinking) functions of the brain

When Stress Becomes Chronic

Sometimes stress is ongoing, and nothing you do seems to help. When stress reduction does not relieve feelings of depression or anxiety, it may be time to seek professional help. You may have *clinical* depression or anxiety. What are the signs of clinical depression or anxiety? They include[22,23]

- Feelings of sadness or anxiety that last for 2 weeks or more
- Chronic exaggerated worry or tension
- Episodes of panic that include physical symptoms such as chest pain, shaking, and trembling that can't be explained by physical reasons
- Flashbacks to traumatic events and nightmares
- Exaggerated startle reactions
- Feelings of hopelessness
- Decreased energy or loss of interest in hobbies and activities you once enjoyed
- Difficulty in staying focused, remembering, or making decisions
- Sleeplessness or oversleeping
- No desire to eat or weight loss or eating to "feel better" and weight gain
- Thoughts of hurting yourself or death or suicide
- Being easily annoyed, bothered, or angered

If these symptoms last for 2 weeks or more, it may be time to consult with your clinician.

The good news is that both anxiety and depression can be treated successfully with a combination of "talk" therapy or psychotherapy and antidepressant and antianxiety medications. If you feel that you do have clinical depression or anxiety, it's important to reach out for help. Talk to your healthcare provider, a trusted friend, or a family member. Don't go it alone—there's help available for those who need it.

Resources for Stress Reduction, Anxiety, and Depression

For more information on stress, anxiety, and depression, try these resources:

Web sites

American Institute of Stress: www.stress.org
American Psychiatric Association: www.psych.org
American Psychological Association: www.apa.org
Anxiety Disorders Association of America: www.adaa.org
National Alliance on Mental Illness: www.nami.org

Books

Benson H, Stark M. *Timeless Healing: the Power and Biology of Belief.* New York: Fireside; 1996.
Burns DD. *Feeling Good: The New Mood Therapy Revised and Updated.* New York: Harper; 1999.
Kabat-Zinn J. *Full Catastrophe Living: Using the Wisdom of Your Body and Mind to Face Stress, Pain, and Illness.* New York: Delacorte Press; 1990.
Manassee Buell L. *Panic and Anxiety Disorder: 121 Tips, Real-life Advice, Resources and More,* 2nd ed. Poway, CA: Simplify Life; 2003.

References

1. Bergelt C, Prescott E, Gronbaek M. Stressful life events and cancer risk. *Br J Cancer.* 2006;95:1579–1581.

2. Nielsen NR. Gronbaek M. Stress and breast cancer: a systematic update on the current knowledge. *Nat Clin Pract Oncol.* 2006;3:612–620.

3. Schraub S, Sancho-Garnier H, Velten M. Should psychological events be considered cancer risk factors. *Rev Epidemiol Sante Publique.* 2009;57:113–123.

4. Garssen B. Psychological factors and cancer development: evidence after 30 years of research. *Clin Psychol Rev.* 2004;24:315–338.

5. National Cancer Institute. *Psychological Stress and Cancer: Questions and Answers.* Available at www.cancer.gov/cancertopics/factsheet/risk/stress. Accessed August 25, 2009.

6. American Cancer Society. *When Someone You Know Has Cancer. General Questions and Answers.* Available at www.cancer.org/docroot/MIT/content/ MIT_1_4x_General_Questions_and_Answers.asp?sitearea=MIT. Accessed August 25, 2009.

7. Schwarz S, Messerschmidt H, Doren M. Psychosocial risk factors for cancer development. *Med Klin.* 2007;102:967–979.

8. Bleiker E, Hendriks J, Otten J, et al. Personality factors and breast cancer risk: a 13-year follow-up. *J Natl Cancer Inst.* 2008;100:213–218.

9. Coyne JC, Pajak TF, Harris J, et al. Emotional well-being does not predict survival in head and neck cancer patients. *Cancer.* 2007;110:2568–2575.

10. Rabin C, Rogers ML, Pinto BM, et al. Effect of personal cancer history and family cancer history and levels of psychological distress. *Soc Sci Med.* 2007;64:411–416.

11. American Cancer Society. *Meditation.* Available at www.cancer.org/docroot/ ETO/content/ETO_5_3X_Meditation.asp. Accessed August 25, 2009.

12. Benson H, Stark M. *Timeless Healing: The Power and Biology of Belief.* New York: Fireside; 1996.

13. American Academy of Family Physicians, FamilyDoctor.org. *Stress: How to Cope Better with Life's Challenges.* Available at familydoctor.org/online/fam-docen/home/common/mentalhealth/stress/167.html. Accessed August 25, 2009.

14. Lance Armstrong Foundation, Livestrong.org. *Stress: Detailed Information.* Available at www.livestrong.org/site/c.khLXK1PxHmF/b.2660711/k.6897/ Emotional_Effects_Stress.htm#d. Accessed August 25, 2009.

15. National Comprehensive Cancer Network. *Clinical Practice Guidelines in Oncology. Distress Management.* Available at www.nccn.org/professionals/ physician_gls/f_guidelines.asp. Accessed August 26, 2009.

16. National Women's Health Information Center Fact Sheet. *Stress and Your Health.* Available at www.womenshealth.gov.

17. American Psychological Association. *Health and Emotional Wellness Fact Sheets. Exercise Fuels the Brain's Stress Buffers.* Available at http://www. apa.org/helpcenter/exercise-stress.aspx. Accessed August 26, 2009.

18. National Center for Complementary and Alternative Medicine. *Yoga for Health: An Introduction.* Available at http://nccam.nih.gov/health/yoga/. Accessed August 27, 2009.

19. National Center for Complementary and Alternative Medicine. *Tai Chi: An Introduction.* Available at http://nccam.nih.gov/health/taichi/. Accessed August 27, 2009.

20. Boughton B. "Relax Your Way to Good Health." *In Touch Magazine*. 2000.

21. National Center for Complementary and Alternative Medicine. *Meditation for Health Purposes*. Available at http://nccam.nih.gov/health/meditation/. Accessed August 27, 2009.

22. National Women's Health Information Center. *Depression: Frequently Asked Questions*. Available at http://womenshealth.gov/faq/depression.cfm. Accessed September 1, 2009.

23. Substance Abuse and Mental Health Services Administration, National Mental Health Information Center. *Anxiety Disorders Fact Sheet*. Available at http://mentalhealth.samhsa.gov/publications/allpubs/ken98–0045/default. asp. Accessed September 1, 2009.

Conclusion
Putting It All Together

A Professional View by Michael Stefanek

A Game Plan for the Future

There is no way to absolutely prevent cancer. However, there is a lot you can do to decrease your risk of developing cancer and detect it early so that your chance of surviving longer with a high quality of life is increased. In this book we have tried our best to provide everything you might want to know about reducing your risk for cancer—at least for now.

As we have mentioned, the science changes, and research may add new information in the future about risk factors discussed in this book. There may be new evidence that comes to light about which factors increase or decrease your risk of developing cancer. Certainly, there will be new ways of screening for cancer developed over time. However, we like to believe that the strengths of this book are that we've included what we know *now* about cancer risk based on the science to date, *and* we've explained how to understand the numbers you might hear when experts and others talk about the risk of cancer as they surface in the future, *and* we've added information on where you might go for dependable advice, with a listing of many Web sites throughout these pages.

You now have lots of information on screening for cancers—which cancers we can effectively screen for, whether you should get screened based on such factors as age and family history, and where to look for additional information about screening. Vigilance to these early detection methods may involve some fear and anxiety about the procedures themselves or worries about the outcome. Yet cancer screening, at least for now, involves at most choosing a behavior on a once-a-year basis.

Although it is critical for the early detection of cancer, screening does not involve behavior change on a *daily* basis, which most people find a very challenging task. Yet the behaviors that decrease the risk of actually developing cancer involve behaviors we participate in daily—including how much we eat, what we eat, how much activity we engage in, and whether or not we smoke. We need to not only initiate change but also to turn our behavior changes into a habit.

If you would like to change the type or amount of food you eat, or increase your physical activity, or stop smoking, we have lots of studies that tell us just how hard it is to *maintain* such behavior change. We know that many people who are ultimately *successful* at stopping smoking often make four to five *unsuccessful* attempts before leaving tobacco behind. Most of us are also very familiar with the "battle of the bulge," and, for every newspaper ad we see claiming, "I lost 50 pounds in 3 days!!!" there are many attempts that fail (not to mention, as in this ad, the number of people who take unhealthy approaches and lose too many pounds too fast). Ditto for exercise. Having been a member of a variety of health clubs over the years, I am very familiar with the "New Year's rush," when, for the first 4 to 5 weeks after New Year's, the health clubs are overrun by those starting out the year determined once and for all to get healthy. Unfortunately, by the end of February, the numbers diminish, and the huge majority of those attempting to change their behavior simply cannot maintain their trips to the treadmill.

We know that there may be societal forces and policies that make it challenging to change our behavior. We are overloaded with ads for high-calorie foods, or perhaps our neighborhoods lack sidewalks for safe walking. Fighting these barriers is not easy. Given how complicated behavior change can be, how can we maintain the drive and determination to really change our behavior? How can we keep our resolve to increase our chances of staying cancer-free and enjoy all the benefits of a healthier lifestyle? Is it simply a matter of willpower? I would agree with Michael Mahoney, a psychologist who wrote a terrific little book back in the late 1970s (*Self Change: Strategies for Solving Personal Problems*) and who does not view willpower as the answer. Dr. Mahoney, at the time, was publishing and writing quite a bit on self-control and personal development and produced this very underutilized book about how to take a step-by-step approach to changing behavior. Although this book, by its title, seems to focus on "personal problems," it applies very well to behavior change overall, and I will review some of the strategies he notes in this classic publication.

So is it all about willpower? No, it is not. There is a myth that says that those who succeed in changing their behavior—losing weight, starting and maintaining an exercise program, stopping smoking—have some magical talent at willing themselves to accomplish these feats. They were blessed with self-control or simply were "stronger" than those who failed. We now know that changing behavior in a healthy direction has more to do with "skillpower"—that is, knowing yourself and your patterns and what works for *you* in changing *your* behavior—not simply "willing" yourself to success. Determination is essential but not enough.

So let me provide an approach that may be helpful as you attempt not only to *begin* behavior change but to *maintain* it—a much more challenging task. This approach is based on what most of us know: We usually do not learn from our own mistakes. We tend to feel a bit annoyed with ourselves for our behavior, set unrealistic goals, and charge ahead boldly in a very determined manner. When our (poorly conceived) plan fails, we become depressed, and our valiant efforts to change our behavior fall short. We may at some point make the same resolution to "get healthy" and dive in again, perhaps this time with a slightly different plan, with the same determination, only to fail again. Rather than put ourselves through this frustrating cycle, let's take a look at a systematic way to change our behavior.

Changing Your Behavior: Steps to Success

S—Specify the behavior to be changed.
C—Collect information.
I—Identify possible causes.
E—Examine possible solutions.
N—Narrow solutions and try.
C—Compare your progress.
E—Extend, revise, or replace your solutions.

Pretty catchy, huh? Yes, *SCIENCE* is a way to remember the steps of behavior change, drawn from the work of Dr. Michael Mahoney mentioned earlier. This acronym takes you from the decision to change your behavior to trying and tweaking your strategies until you find a successful solution. Let's go over each step so that you have a solid sense of how to develop your "skillpower" to more fully engage in healthy behavior.

Specify

The first step is to define the problem. This is the easiest step at all, especially because we're talking only about behaviors that influence our cancer risk. This could be anything from increasing your physical activity, to losing weight, to eating healthier, or to giving up smoking—behaviors that you may engage in on a frequent basis.

In setting up a specific behavior change, you should consider both short- and long-term goals. The former might involve goals for the next few weeks, whereas the latter would be more remote. The short-term goals are actually the most critical because they not only move you toward your long-term objectives but also give you an early sign about barriers and problems you might face and help to keep you motivated.

Your goals also should be realistic. If you are a 55-year-old, you may want to keep your goals a notch below what you see from those 20-year-olds at the gym. Although goals can be very helpful, they can be disastrous if you set goals that are too perfectionist or unreasonable. If you have any doubts about how reasonable your goals are, you might check with family members or friends for their thoughts. What else should you keep in mind? Consider the following as you set your goals:

- Try to make a change that is fairly small and comfortable at first.
- Frame the goal in terms of *doing* something rather than *not doing* something (e.g., eating more vegetables versus not eating as much red meat).
- Try to select behaviors that have the active encouragement and support of your family members and friends.
- Select modest changes that are slowly increased over time (walk one-half mile before running a mile).

Collect Information

Getting accurate information about your behavior before starting to change is critical for a program's success. It shows you where you have been and, over time, how far you have advanced. As Michael Mahoney notes, "It is hard to get directions if you don't know where you are."

You need to decide what information is helpful to gather. Perhaps you grab a cigarette after you are stressed or when you feel depressed, so tracking what happens before grabbing a cigarette or how you feel when you do so might be important information. Other information also may be helpful: What time is it? Who is present? Where am I? I know ex-smokers who always smoked on the phone, so knowing this strong link to this unhealthy behavior was very important to them in crafting a strategy to stop.

It is important to write this information down soon after it happens so that memory is not an issue. It is also crucial to track this information for about 10 days before you begin your program so that you have an excellent sample of the behavior you want to change. This allows you to get through at least one weekend and allows you to be sure that you are tracking all the important information needed. It also allows you to get used to recording the information—which you will continue once you start your program. It is very easy to get impatient and want to get your program started immediately—but remember once again, "It is hard to get directions if you don't know where you are."

Identify Possible Causes

All of us get wrapped up in wondering "why" we do something, and we can get lost in theories, hunches, and "psychobabble." It is more helpful to ask "when" or "how" we indulge in a behavior. If you insist on asking "why," then the answers to "when" and "how" can provide a more informed answer. Most psychologists are aware of the ABCs of behavior. Although "B" is the behavior, "A" is the antecedent, or what happens before the behavior, and "C" is the consequence, or what happens after. Both can influence our behavior. If I am trying to stop eating ice cream, putting me in the ice cream aisle at the local supermarket (the "A") is likely to increase my ice cream buying. If I reward my walks into the kitchen with ice cream during a commercial, my walks are rewarded with a tasty treat (the "C").

Although we have been talking mostly about situations and people related to your behavior, you also have to realize the importance of thoughts, feelings, and images. You may need to increase the number of times you say something positive to yourself after engaging in a healthy behavior to reinforce it—and don't wait until you finish the behavior to do so! If you have a hard time making that turn into the health club parking lot after a hard day's work, congratulate yourself after doing so, and continue to do so as you step onto that treadmill. If you have friends or family members supporting your behavior change, share with them this success at sticking with your workout rather than heading home. You also may hear that unhealthy voice in your head telling you how tired you are, how you can work out tomorrow, etc. Talk back—and tell that voice that you are working out today, or imagine yourself 20 pounds lighter when you reach your long-term goal! Finally, look at the information you have collected over your 10 days. Find patterns that lead to the behavior you are trying to change. If you can't find such a pattern, ask your family members or friends to find one. Since they're a step removed from the program you want to begin, they can help with this "detective" work.

Examine Possible Solutions

After examining the data you have gathered for your behavior-change project, keep in mind thoughts and behaviors and situations that might have influenced the behavior, and consider making changes in as many of these areas as possible. It is often a combination of thoughts ("I am so hungry . . . I really need some ice cream"), situations (being in a grocery store), and behavior (walking over to the ice cream section) that contributes to keeping an unhealthy behavior rolling along. Also, don't worry about coming up with a complete *solution immediately*—rather, focus on making *improvements* in moving your behaviors toward being more consistent with a healthier lifestyle. Of course, there are some behaviors that involve stopping completely, such as smoking or, if drinking is a problem, alcohol intake.

If you have thoughts or beliefs that are getting in the way ("I just can't stop eating ice cream. . . . it is hopeless"), look for holes in your belief system and ways to change your thoughts. Try to think of any times when you did succeed at not eating ice cream—what happened then? Isn't that evidence that you can do it? Just because you have struggled before, does this mean that it is written in stone that ice cream will forever control you?

Here is where you can have fun brainstorming. There are no "right" or "wrong" ways to change your behaviors. The key is, "What has the best chance of working *for you*?" What are all the strategies that you might use to change your behavior? What might you change about your thoughts? How might you change the situations you are in to make behavior change possible? What might your family members or friends be able to do to help? Develop as long a list as possible. Use your imagination at this point, and don't cross anything off your list!

Narrow Your Solutions and Try

So now you have collected information for 10 days or so and have examined patterns, and being a creative person, you've arrived at a dozen possible solutions to how to reduce your cancer risk. Now what? Being successful requires more than just "doing something," so what do you do? First, after listing all possible options, review them to see which ones are really possible. You may have some that are just not possible. Next, cross off those from the list that seem to you to have the least likelihood of working. Do they rely on someone's help who has not been consistent in the past? If so, perhaps it may be best not to use this strategy as a key component of your plan. Are there behavior changes that simply seem like they involve too much work to maintain? Those can be crossed off your list.

Keep working until you come down to your top two to four candidates. Do not pick those that are simply the easiest but rather those that are possible and that have the highest likelihood of succeeding. You might think of combining these in some way that might work. Once you have this list, take a moment and close your eyes and imagine how these solutions might work. Actually imagine yourself in the situation and any barriers that might interfere with its success. If there are barriers, you may need to drop or revise your goals. If there are few hindrances to your behavior changes, ask yourself the following questions as you trim your list:

- Are these solutions realistic—will I really be able to implement my plan?
- Is it really likely to change my behavior?
- What obstacles have I overlooked?
- Is there anything about these solutions that is worse than the problem?
- Is there any way I might revise these solutions to make them even more successful?

If your solutions pass this test, you might just have a winner or two and be on your way to a healthier life.

Compare Your Progress

Stick with your program for 4 to 6 weeks. You really need this much time to see if it is working, what consistent barriers you might find, and how well it compares with your behavior before starting your program. But you need to be flexible. If you encounter an insurmountable barrier to your strategy that you didn't envision beforehand, then certainly you need to be flexible and revise. However, the usual tendency is to stop a program too early—before you can really see how well it is working.

You also need to make sure that you keep records for these first 4 to 6 weeks so that you have solid information as a base to revise your program as needed. This process may seem slow, but think about how long you have been smoking or how long you have been wallowing in physical inactivity or carrying too much weight around. You cannot change a behavior overnight that has perhaps taken years to settle in place.

So how do you know if your program is working? Keep in mind that we are looking for improvements, not perfection. You may not arrive at your ultimate goal in 4 to 6 weeks, but if you are *moving* in the right direction, stick with it! You also may notice trends over 4 to 6 weeks. Perhaps, after a dismal start, the program really kicks in during weeks 4 to 6. If you had stopped it after week 2, you would have given up on a very promising strategy. Finally, look for any changes in your behavior. Do you now smoke in more limited situations? Do you eat high-calorie dishes less often but really load up when you do eat them? Are there certain friends who are being even more supportive than expected and others who may need a prompt? It may be an overused cliché, but it is critical to remember "the journey of a thousand miles starts with the first step."

Extend, Revise, or Replace

Try to avoid labeling your behavior-change attempt as a "failure" or a "success." It is rare to have a perfect success the first time around (although we hope that you are an exception). Thus you can always "tweak" your strategies to strengthen them. Alternatively, it is not possible for your attempt to be a total failure unless you have learned *nothing at all* about what makes your behavior change difficult. If you have had some degree of success in reaching your goal, congratulations! It is now time to continue the strategy and see how well it maintains the behavior. You may now track the behavior every second or third week rather than every week, just to make sure that there is no slippage. If there is, go back to daily tracking to solve the mystery of why the program has stopped working. Gradually, as you feel that the new behavior has truly become a "habit" and part of your daily living, you can decide to stop tracking it totally, coming back to it only if you notice your weight going up, cigarette cravings increasing, pants getting a bit snug around the waist, or vegetables and/or fruit disappearing from your menu or you realize that your turn into the health club parking lot is getting much more difficult to maneuver.

On the other hand, if your program simply was not as successful as you had hoped, you might review the following questions suggested by Dr. Mahoney:

- Are you confident in the accuracy of the information you gathered during the program?
- Did you allow sufficient time to evaluate the program?
- Were there any unforeseen circumstances or situations that would have kept virtually any strategy from working during the time you put the program into effect?
- Are you confident that you have examined all possible signs of improvement?

If you answer "Yes" to all of these questions and the program did not work, you might go back to the data-collection phase with your knowledge of what barriers you experienced, and what did not work. The goal would be to revise your program and start anew with record collection. You also might enlist a "life coach," now popular in a variety of communities, or a behavioral therapist, typically a psychologist who specializes in behavior change, often found by contacting your state's psychological association. If increasing your physical activity is the goal, a personal trainer from a community health club might be helpful. Again, keep the goal of improvement, not perfection, in mind. Losing weight, increasing physical activity, and eating healthier are all positive changes, even if you do not meet your planned goals in any of these areas. In the case of tobacco, see Chapter 6 for a host of valuable resources, including quitlines, counseling, and medications.

Finally, remember that most of us do not succeed the first time, and many of us don't make it even the second or third time. If we learn something about ourselves and what keeps our unhealthy behavior maintained with each attempt, we are likely on our way to eventual success!

So now you have a lot of information about reducing your cancer risk. You also have the ability to head into the future armed with ways to evaluate information you receive about cancer risk. As you have read, there *are* ways to reduce your cancer risk, and many of these also decrease your risk of other health problems.

Benjamin Franklin once said that two things in life are inevitable— death and taxes. You notice that he did not say "cancer." We agree with Ben.

Take care. We wish you a long, healthy, happy life.

Appendix
Evaluating Scientific Evidence

Evaluating Evidence and Claims About
Cancer Risk and Prevention

If you read Chapter 1, "What Is Cancer Risk," then you already know quite a bit about interpreting the numbers that are used (and misused) in explaining cancer risk and cancer prevention. In this Appendix we're going to consider where those numbers come from, which will help you to understand which numbers (and which conclusions, claims, or promises) you read and hear are believable and relevant to you. In some cases, the conclusions and numbers will be based on very strong evidence. In others, the evidence may be very preliminary or flawed. And sometimes the evidence presented to you (especially in advertisements and on the Internet) may be intentionally distorted or even made up.[1]

Preclinical Studies

Preclinical studies (which do not involve human participants) have an important role in cancer research. In general, human studies are undertaken only when test tube studies or laboratory animal studies indicate that a new treatment is likely to be safe and effective in humans. Unfortunately, these preclinical studies are not even close to perfect in predicting clinical safety and benefit, so it is generally unwise to base health decisions entirely on their results. There are some exceptions, though. For example, it's generally wise to avoid or minimize exposure to anything that causes cancer in animals, unless there is strong evidence to believe that these animal studies are not relevant to humans.

Human Studies

One of the weakest forms of evidence is the **testimonial**, or claims of one person. In some ways, basing decisions on one or even a few testimonials is like flipping a coin once. If you flipped a coin 100 times and got 100 tails, you could be very confident that you have a coin with tails on both sides. Even if you got 80 tails, you could confidently suspect there is something unusual about your coin. But flipping the coin once or even a few times tells you almost nothing. Likewise, knowing a few smokers who lived to age 90 and never developed cancer tells you only that some smokers don't develop cancer. It tells you almost nothing about how smoking affects a person's risk of developing cancer (see Chapter 6 for more information on smoking).

The same limitations apply to factors suspected of reducing cancer risk. Anecdotal reports of good or bad outcomes of someone who ate lots of a certain food, took a particular supplement, or followed some other cancer-prevention plan are almost useless, even assuming that that the person's story is accurate (and we'll say more about that later on).

There are several kinds of studies that use information from more than one person (and usually from many more) to make conclusions about factors that increase or decrease cancer risk.

Ecological studies look for correlations between diseases such as cancer and risk factors or protective factors in groups of people. What distinguishes these studies from some other kinds of research is that the scientists do not collect information about individuals in the group but only about aggregate characteristics of the group. For example, an ecological study might compare diet and cancer risk in the United States and China. One result would be that Chinese people have lower cancer risk and drink more tea. Although this result suggests that tea might be beneficial, this is extremely weak evidence because the low cancer risk in China also might be due to less obesity, more exercise, less meat, or a number of equally plausible factors. This kind of study also can be used to suggest correlations that don't make much sense when you delve deeper. Although speaking Chinese is correlated with lower cancer risk, if an overweight, sedentary American smoker wanted to lower his or her cancer risk, taking a course to learn the Chinese language would not be at the top of our list of recommendations.

Case-control studies compare risk factors or protective factors in two groups of people—cases, who have a disease such as cancer, and controls, who do not. Most case-control studies are retrospective, meaning that participants are asked about past exposure to risk factors or protective factors. So one problem is that many people don't accurately recall what they ate years ago or how much they exercised or what medi-cines they took. Another problem is that sometimes the cases (people with the disease) put more effort into trying to accurately recall their past exposures; this undermines the accuracy of the study. Or if the cases are already very sick, they may be less able to accurately recall their past. Even worse, if the cases are already suspicious that something (perhaps chemicals in their workplace or neighborhood) may have caused their cancer, they may subconsciously overestimate their past exposures. There are many other ways, which you could read about in epidemiology books, for case-control studies to go awry. Overall, these studies can be very useful when they are conducted thoroughly, but they are not perfect and need to be interpreted with caution.

Cohort studies start with a large group of healthy volunteers and collect information about risk factors or protective factors. Because researchers record this information before some members of the cohort develop the disease in question, these are also **prospective** studies. Since these studies take place in real time, they avoid problems with inaccurate recall of risk factors or protective factors and generally provide stronger evidence than **retrospective** case-control studies.

But both case-control studies and cohort studies can have other problems owing to effects of factors not recorded and analyzed by the researchers. Let's consider a hypothetical study of whether dryclean-ing solvents (see Chapter 9 for more information) might increase cancer death rates. And let's imagine that the researchers compared people who wear drycleaned clothing at least five times per week with people who rarely or never do. A simple study of these two factors probably would suggest that wearing drycleaned clothing reduces your risk of dying from cancer. The problem is that this imaginary study neglected to consider other differences between the people who often or rarely/never have their clothes drycleaned. People who wear drycleaned clothing often are likely to be wearing suits to work. They are likely to work indoors at occupa-tions that do not involve exposure to industrial or agricultural chemicals. They are likely to be relatively affluent and educated and to be nonsmok-ers, and they probably have good health insurance. In an actual study, epidemiologists probably would use mathematical methods to control for some of these differences. But, unless they recognized and collected data on the most important differences, their conclusions still could be distorted—a problem known as *uncontrolled confounding*.

Clinical trials are studies in which volunteers agree to receive a particular therapy so that researchers can learn whether it is safe and effective. Although most people think of clinical trials as ways to test new drugs for people who already have cancer, clinical trials also can test ways to prevent or diagnose disease or to relieve symptoms, and they may not involve any drugs (some clinical trials test special diets, exercise programs, medical devices, operations, etc.).

In *nonrandomized* clinical trials, all participants receive the new treatment. These trials are very important as early studies on the safety and effectiveness of new cancer treatments, especially when there is concern that the treatment may have serious side effects or may not work at all. Although they also have a role in cancer prevention, in this discussion we will concentrate on *randomized* clinical trials because they can avoid most of the pitfalls of ecological, case-control, and cohort studies and therefore can provide the most convincing evidence regarding cancer prevention.

In general, randomized clinical trials (RCTs) are considered the "gold standard" in research. In **randomized clinical trials,** participants are randomly assigned to receive a new treatment or some other treatment and/or sometimes no treatment at all; for example, one group may be started on a special low-fat diet, with the other group continuing their usual diet. Some randomized trials compare a medication or supplement (such as a vitamin or mineral) versus an inactive pill called a *placebo*. Because the researchers assign the treatment, there is no problem with inaccurate recall, as in a retrospective study. And assigning the treatments randomly usually avoids concerns about other differences between the two groups being compared.

Although clinical trials are very important in evaluating strategies for cancer prevention, there are obvious ethical limitations. Of course, it would not be ethical to intentionally expose people to known or suspected carcinogens. For this reason, most of our understanding of cancer risk factors is based on animal studies and studies of people exposed to carcinogens accidentally, unknowingly (in unsafe workplaces, for example) or by their own choice (for example, smoking).

It also would be unethical to withhold something of known benefit. For example, it is possible to conduct a clinical trial comparing a control group eating their usual diet versus a group encouraged to eat more vegetables and fruits, but it would be unethical to include a group of people asked to stop eating vegetables and fruits.

Reference

1. Ades T, Gansler T, Alteri R. *American Cancer Society's Complete Guide to Complementary and Alternative Cancer Methods*, 2nd ed. New York: American Cancer Society; 2009.

Index